D0374213

SCIENCE
MEETS
ALTERNATIVE MEDICINE

SCIENCE
MEETS
ALTERNATIVE MEDICINE

*What the Evidence Says
About Unconventional Treatments*

edited by

Wallace Sampson, M.D.,
& Lewis Vaughn

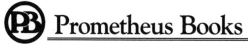 Prometheus Books

59 John Glenn Drive
Amherst, New York 14228-2197

Published 2000 by Prometheus Books

Inquiries should be addressed to
Prometheus Books
59 John Glenn Drive
Amherst, New York 14228–2197
VOICE: 716–691–0133, ext. 207
FAX: 716–564–2711
WWW.PROMETHEUSBOOKS.COM

04 03 02 01 00   5 4 3 2 1

Library of Congress Cataloging-in-Publication Data

Science meets alternative medicine : what the evidence says about unconventional
    treatments / edited by Wallace Sampson and Lewis Vaughn.
        p. cm.
    Includes bibliographical references.
    ISBN 1–57392–803–8 (pbk.)
    1. Alternative medicine. 2. Evidence. I. Sampson, Wallace. II. Vaughn, Lewis.

R733 .S38   2000
615.5—dc21   00–023169
                                                                              CIP

Printed in the United States of America on acid-free paper

CONTENTS

THERAPIES AND THEORIES

ETHICS, FRAUD, AND RISKS

INTRODUCTION

Wallace Sampson

A T LEAST THREE DECADES HAVE PASSED AS INTEREST HAS INCREASED IN more ancient, native, and sometimes bizarre medical customs. This phenomenon, the interest in anomalous methods now known as "alternative medicine," has caused the commercial community to act. It lobbies for law changes and invents new questionably effective products and remarkably effective marketing methods. Academics, the press, and the plain curious ask why? Why now?

The answer, as with any major social movement, lies in a complex of factors, happening to coalesce "now" in the 1980s and 90s. Not the least are the constant interests of a segment of the population in returning to the mysterious and spiritual nature of prescientific medicine. Those people and others have personal but natural tendencies to counter authority, to seek explanations for events and complex matters not easily understood, to confuse causes and effects, and otherwise misinterpret events. Or may just possess a large genetic dose of natural gullibility.

Behind the constant reasons are two twentieth-century academic developments. First is cultural relativism, which equates primitive, empirical, ineffective methods with those of proved effectiveness for the sake of being nonjudgmental of others' customs. The other is postmodernism, which dismisses the importance of validity in pursuit of its casuistry that denies facts and the very existence of a rationally discernable external reality.

Two practical factors make it all happen. The presence of billions of dollars in grant money from wealthy foundations pays for the research, academic positions, and journals, and for expensive television productions and conferences. The peculiar journalistic ethic or principle of balance and objectivity dictates that reporters present absurd medical concepts and behavior as if they were just different in some minor ways from standards based on rationality and science. Without the infusion from wealthy ideologues and a gullible and complementary press, the public would find it difficult to know of the existence of most aberrant medical methods.

But there is even more operating to propel the wave of interest and acceptance. I mentioned gullibility. Manipulating the public's essentially trusting nature is a concerted effort on the part of "alternative" advocates to obscure their real nature and intent, and to present their wares falsely. That is the most shocking of the forces behind the movement, and is one that, of course, will be vigorously denied. But the evidence is clear, as illustrated by the intentional misuse and distortion of language ("alternative," "unorthodox," "unconventional," to describe ineffective methods and quackery), and the repetitive use of false medical myths and propaganda slogans (medicine is reductionist, only 10 percent of standard methods are proved, doctors only "cut, burn, and poison"). Even the famous surveys of the popular use of aberrant methods were conceived and reported inaccurately to fulfill the advocates' prophesies. These matters were explored at the conference.

The Committee for Scientific Investigation of Claims of the Paranormal and the *Scientific Review of Alternative Medicine*, aided by the Mclean Contributorship of Philadelphia organized this first major North American program, to explore this peculiar movement. We gathered experts on psychology, medicine, physics, chemistry, pharmacology, philosophy, and ethics in a forum to explore and explain all of this heady stuff. We were honored by the presence of three guest speakers, all distinguished present or past editors of major medical journals, Marcia Angell, M.D., George Lundberg, M.D., and Arnold Relman, M.D.

The journal *SRAM* and many books published by Prometheus Books offer more in-depth commentary and analysis than can be presented in this volume. But for this introduction to the world of aberrant medicine and anomalous claims, the conference presenters have performed a major public service. When this odd episode of human events is examined two hundred years from now, I hope historians will recognize the contents as islands of rationality in this storm of lost bearings. The presenters' contents need not be reviewed here, since the presentations are understandable and pointed. Readers will want to proceed rapidly to their main course, for many tasty moments of revelation and appetizing thoughts for stimulating discussion. We at CSICOP, *SRAM*, and Prometheus are indebted to the presenters for their generous contributions. We hope you will enjoy reading their remarks as we enjoyed hearing them in Philadelphia.

ORIGINS
AND
TRENDS

1

IN DEFENSE OF
SCIENTIFIC MEDICINE

Paul Kurtz

I

THE PUBLIC IS BEING INUNDATED BY NEW AGE SPIRITUALISTIC THERAPIES. Pseudoscientific health cures are highly popular in the media and among book and magazine publishers—visit any bookstore today and compare the shelf space devoted to science books with New Age, Occult, or Paranormal books.

As skeptics, we have encouraged research by the scientific community into these paranormal claims and we have published criticism of them. One question that is often asked by the media and the general public is this: Why should anyone bother to criticize clairvoyance, astrology, phrenology, or numerology? What harm do these do? Aren't they fun? In the past we would immediately respond by referring to blatant quackery in the health area—from faith heating by evangelical hucksters to Edgar Cayce's diagnosis of disease and his alleged cures. The uncritical public acceptance of health fads and diets can be dangerous to the public's health, especially if people substitute these nostrums for competent medical treatment. When we began our skeptical agenda, little did we imagine that alternative or complementary medicine would grow as rapidly as it has, especially in the past decade.

The National Institute of Health established an Office of Alternative

Medicine in 1992 is funded with federal dollars, and there are many new alternative-medicine journals. Many of its leading doctor-gurus, such as Deepak Chopra, Andrew Wed, Bernie Siegal, and Larry Dossey, have published best-selling books that dominate the public's perception of medicine. Moreover, as Marcia Angell and Jerome P. Kassiter, editors of the *New England Journal of Medicine*, point out (September 17, 1998) the multibillion-dollar "dietary-supplement industry" is now exempt from Federal Food and Drug Administration (FDA) regulation; and the public isinundated with advertising claims. The Dietary-Supplement Health and Education Act, which was enacted in 1994, allows herbal remedies to be sold without requiring the manufacturer to prove their effectiveness and safety to the FDA. According to a recent story in the *New York Times* (February 1999), a federal judge ordered the FDA to lift its ban on cholestin, a powder made from a Chinese rice fermented with red yeast. The Agency had banned the import of this unapproved drug, which had been marketed as a dietary supplement. The powder contains a natural form of lovastatin, which is a key ingredient in Mevacor, a cholesterolreducing prescription drug.

Alternative medicine is growing also because many health-maintenance organizations and insurance companies now cover alternative medicine treatments. According to the *Wall Street Journal* (February 18, 1999), practitioners of the ancient art of healing known as Reiki won't need a license to practice their craft. The New York Massage Board voted to allow them to go unlicensed. Reiki masters allegedly heal with "spiritual energy" that flows through their hands without touching their patients. Ellen Kahne of New York City, according to the journal, claims that she was able to stop her cousin's asthma attack, even though hundreds of miles away! In response to the growth of public interest in alternative medicine, many medical schools are now teaching courses in it. We thus are suddenly faced with the extraordinary growth of alternative therapies, often in competition with scientific medicine.

With this problem in mind, many of us associated with the skeptics movement decided to organize a systematic response to alternative medicine. Thus we created in late 1997 an informal *ad hoc* "Council for Scientific Medicine," and we launched a new peer-reviewed journal, the *Scientific Review of Alternative Medicine*. In my view, the American Medical Association should have organized such a group, but ever since the chiropractic profession successfully sued the AMA, that association has been reluctant to get into the fray. They are at times more concerned with their professional prerogatives than their social responsibilities. Because they have not entered into the fray, we have taken the initiative in organizing this effort.

The goal of the Council for Scientific Medicine is to defend the integrity and the importance of scientific medicine. Health has always been of primary concern to human beings—fearful of disease, pain, suffering, and death, they seek relief. Medical cures were based historically on folk medicine, cultural traditions, and religious superstitions. These remedies no doubt had some basis in experience, but cures were not grounded on rigorously tested knowledge and were often unreliable. A good illustration of a folk cure is as follows:

> My oldest brother had a toothache, and a man told us: You know them places that be on the inside of a mule's leg looks like it been sore or something. He told us to get a pocket knife and trim some of that off and put it in a pipe and let my brother smoke it. And we did that, and it stopped it.[1]

Everyone knows that grandmother's chicken soup is an excellent remedy for a cold, and that it will relieve symptoms in one week. Of course, without grandma's chicken soup it would take seven days. Folk medicine historically consisted basically of the use of vegetable products or herbs, or various forms of diet and exercise, some of these are no doubt effective, many of them based on the placebo effect. China and India and other Asian countries have a long history of traditional medicine. CSICOP had exchanged delegations with China, and we have visited institutes for Traditional Chinese Medicine in Beijing and Shanghai. One illustration of Chinese folk cures dramatically points to the problem. While in Beijing, James Alcock, a member of our first skeptics delegation to China in 1988, developed a bad cough and he went to a Chinese clinic, which offered to provide him with snake bile. The question we asked was, "Does it work or not?" Of course, the only way to tell is by rigorous testing. Alcock decided not to take it and managed to get some antibiotics.

II

In any case, scientific medicine is a relatively recent development in human history, especially in the nineteenth century, when increased knowledge of physiology and human anatomy was refined. There have been a number of brilliant researchers who have contributed to our understanding, such as Claude Bernard, the French scientist, who used experimental methods to clarify the role of the pancreas and of glycogen in the liver. There have been great breakthroughs in microbiology and bacteriology with the introduction of germ and bacteria theories by Louis Pasteur, Robert Koch, and others. The discovery of the importance of antiseptics was demonstrated by Joseph Lister. Theories about the nature and transmission of infectious disease, such as diphtheria, tuberculosis, yellow fever, malaria, typhoid, tetanus, polio, and the development of vaccines all had important roles in immunization. Likewise important were the great advances in epidemiology, public health, and sanitation. In the twentieth century endocrinology advanced—with the discovery of insulin, cortisone, and sex hormones. In the field of nutrition researchers discovered the important role of vitamins. There have been significant new diagnostic tools, such as X-ray imagery, CT scans, and mammography and sonograms. The great strides in surgery have been impressive, including cardiology, neurosurgery, and organ transplantation. The discovery of antibiotics has made enormous contributions to the cure of infectious disease. We should add to this the discoveries of DNA, biogenetic research, gene therapy, and other innovations on the frontiers of research. All of these achievements have led to the reduction of infant mortality and the extension of life spans—over three decades have been added to longevity rates in the twentieth century in affluent countries. As part of this process was the development, beginning in 1904, of rigorous standards of medical education in medical schools. Thus we see the remarkable effectiveness of modern scientific medicine—all for the benefit of humankind.

The question can be raised: How does scientific medicine relate to alternative medicine? Our response is that we should apply the same rigorous peer-review process to the claims of alternative medical proponents. What does this entail? First, that practitioners of alternative medicine have a coherent, clearly defined explanatory theory that is internally consistent and falsifiable. We are concerned that acupuncture, chiropractic, chigong, and therapeutic touch, for example, lack such identifiable theories. Second, at the very least therapeutic practices and medications need to be rigorously tested. Here we are not talking about anecdotal information, hearsay, or self-proclaimed validations by their practitioners, but independent corroboration, double-blind, randomized, controlled clinical tests. We need statistical evidence of the reliability of such cures before we can accept them.

There is an ongoing battle between the advocates of scientific medicine and their critics. Many New Age alternative healers deny that science is applicable. They denigrate the medical establishment. They believe that skeptics dogmatically reject unconventional therapies. They think that there are hidden untapped powers of ancient natural remedies and therapies that need to be released.

Skeptics should not seek to defend the medical profession per se. Medical doctors are practical craftsmen, drawing on intuition and their own experience, and some perhaps are not sufficiently familiar with the methods of scientific research. The so-called medical establishment has in the past opposed novel theories and important pioneers, such as Pasteur and Simmelweis, who had to battle against received doctrines.

The medical profession has suffered two waves of criticism in the last thirty years. First, in the late 1960s and early 1970s the field of medical ethics developed. This sought to dethrone authoritarian doctors and to defend the rights of patients. The euthanasia movement is a dramatic illustration of this development; so is the demand for informed choice and the right of patients to resist treatment. After some controversy, medical ethics was accepted by those within the medical community, who, along with philosophers, ethicists, theologians, lawyers and the lay public, have developed new ethical guidelines for treatment. Second, alternative medicine now challenges the medical profession. It seems to me that the only adequate response is to be open to new claims of therapy, provided they are responsibly framed and testable. Thus we need to evaluate such claims and to seek to have them corroborated. We hope this will contribute, in a modest way, to the advancement of medical knowledge—and it should apply to orthodox as well as to alternative medicine.

III

The paradox that we face today is that this assault on scientific medicine is occurring in spite of the extraordinary advances that are being achieved. Why is this so? There are various explanations that I can only briefly suggest.

First, the traditional family doctor is being replaced by HMOs, clinics, and by teams of specialists. Many of these have lost the intimate personal relationship that medical practitioners of the past have had.

Second, hopeless patients in the terminal stages of cancer or other debilitating diseases often give up on orthodox scientific medicine and seek alternative cures. They are desperate to seek some help.

Third, many people swear by alternative medicine because they believe it is effective. This, I think, can be attributed to many factors: Many illnesses of the body, if left alone, will in time heat themselves. There are vague pains and maladies that are undiagnosed and which may in time also dissipate. The placebo effect can be powerful in regard to psychosomatic if not organic illnesses. Medical science is not infallible. There are many diseases we do not understand, nor are cures available. Moreover, the state of the art is constantly changing, and earlier methods subsequently may have to be abandoned or revised. Many patients do not understand the tentative fallible character of the process of scientific inquiry. We need to edify them and especially focus on preventative medicine.

Fourth, alternative medicine has become a highly profitable industry. Food additives, dietary supplements, herbs, and vitamins are being marketed to the public, often with few if any qualifications about their effectiveness. The media-oriented companies that dominate our society often focus on sensationalized reports of miracle therapies, and there has not been a national effort to provide adequate balanced information to the public.

Fifth, the growth of alternative medicine is related to other antiscientific attitudes in society. It is allied with a vague kind of regnant spirituality, especially in the writings of Deepak Chopra and Andrew Weil; and this has an affinity with New Age paradigms. It is also reinformed by postmodern attacks on objectivity in science. If knowledge is ultimately validated subjectively, or by its relationship to a culture, then anecdotal reports and folk medicine would be admissible forms of "validation."

Skepticism has its work cut out for it. For human health is too precious to be squandered by premodern nostrums or postmodern fantasies. We need to submit the claims of health cures to careful evaluation. We need an open mind and should not prejudge the issue before inquiry. We also need to stimulate an appreciation in the public about the nature of scientific medicine and the need for caution about untested remedies.

NOTE

1. Quoted by Frank Reuter in "Folk Remedies and Human Belief-Systems: How Body and Mind Work Together to Make Folk Remedies Seem Successful," *Skeptical Inquirer* 11, no. 1 (fall 1986): 44.

2

THE BRAID OF "ALTERNATIVE MEDICINE"

Wallace Sampson

REPORTERS ASK US, "WHAT ARE THE REASONS FOR THE POPULARITY OF 'alternative medicine' ("AM," or "CAM" for "complementary and alternative medicine")? Why now?"

The question is challenging, the search for answers tantalizing, and the answers difficult to substantiate. Yet the temptation to answer is irresistible. As in a braid, no one factor can explain the whole phenomenon. Some factors are more important than others, some are antecedent, others are more direct and recent, and some feed on others then combine with their antecedents that again operate currently.

PREDISPOSING AND ANTECEDENT SYSTEMS

There are a number of predisposing psychological and political influences. In North America, such influences include a mistrust of government, politicians, highbrows, elitists, professionals, and other authorities. Other factors are deregulation, loss of power of governmental agencies, increasing court awards for perceived injuries, and Internet do-it-yourself medicine.

In Germany, perhaps a key factor is the feeling of unity with Nature (Naturphilosophie) required for action to be complete and satisfying. Add a tint of Hahnemann's homeopathy, Steiner's anthroposophical medicine, and a few mystical legends. In Britain, perhaps it is the tolerance of the unique, eccentric, and bizarre. In Asia, it is the sense of tradition and partnering of spirituality and cosmology with all phases of life.

North Americans are enamored of a melange of folkways from European countries, mixed through the eighteenth and nineteenth centuries into a new brand. Thomson, Kellogg, Post, Graham, and Mary Baker Eddy interpreted and recombined them, and passed them through D. D. Palmer to lack Lalanne, Andrew Weil, and Larry Dossey.

Technical, professional, scientific medicine is about a hundred years old. We separate slowly from folkway methods that stick to common consciousness. We reflect and repeat our parents' quaint ideas and irritating habits. One of my family's holdovers was that fever came from toxins built up in the colon—a notion familiar to turn-of-the-century scholars as one of Kellogg's basic premises, putrefaction. It resulted in the feared, torturous enema, a punishment for having gotten ill.

Then there are customs like wearing of animal fat around the torso and the water cures (soaks and religious purification rites to drive out bad spirits that inhabit warm places). They appeal to those who want to explore the past, hoping to find Answers to Everything in mysteries, then proclaiming them to the unawakened public. These emotional-spiritual undercurrents of need are strong determinants of behavior, say historians and psychologists. We tend to agree.

CULTURAL RELATIVISM

Whether it is an undercurrent or a propelling force (a case could be made for either), the essence of all these threads seems to lead to a loss of standards for thought and action, and a disregard of intellectual discipline.

Cultural relativism was born in the early twentieth century, in the innocence of academic fairness and objectivity. Its intent was to omit prejudice and emotion in the investigation of other cultures. Previously one could read only xenophobic, supercilious descriptions of other cultures, even of our own subcultures. Observers used pejorative terms such as quaint, backward, primitive, pagan, savage. Relativism raised cultural anthropology from biased emotionality of supercultures and superraces to realistic, judgment-free, academically productive understandings. It allowed an appreciation for the healthy diversity of human cultural evolution.

But cultural relativism became inappropriately applied, like using a screwdriver to drive a nail. Relativism was applied to medical systems as if they merely reflected cultural differences instead of being approaches that were more or less useful for increasing health and longevity. judgment-free description of the system replaced the system's objective value to health. In relativistic schemes, the number of days of illness, numbers and sizes of epidemics, mortality rates, life spans, cure rates, misery, and pain are all ignored. The measure of a medical system became how well it helped the culture's functioning and cohesiveness.

This disconnect persists despite scientific data about modem biomedicine's obvious objective benefits. Worthless and harmful traditional remedies are rationalized as being just "different," "alternative," "traditional," "unorthodox." Acupuncture, for example, is rationalized by saying "if it has worked for three thousand years, there must be something to it." But "worked" is never quantitatively defined. Of course, the same could be said for tiger parts used for male potency. Decimation of wild animal species for imagined effects of their parts does enter the perceived benefit equation. Cultural relativism results in this peculiar blindness to folkways' untoward consequences in favor of "nonjudgmental" description.

Reluctance to criticize another culture's medical system through fear of appearing insensitive is now a form of political correctness—a straightjacket of niceness. Traditional-healing advocates demand niceness on threat of accused bias. Yet they demonstrate selfishness and narcissism and closed-mindedness to reason. A man recently proclaimed on an Internet page that his mother's amyotrophic lateral sclerosis improved after a healer waved his hand over hers. When others suggested reasonable alternative explanations for the perceived improvement, the son was incensed that anyone could be so crass and insensitive to the family's cultural tradition as to suggest a misinterpretation of the event. The son could not conceive that others might be adversely affected by false miracles. Nonbelievers had better be nice or be silent.

At the American Association for the Advancement of Science in 1979, sociologists convened a conference on laetrile, a fraudulent cancer remedy. Criminal backgrounds of promoters and the biochemical implausibilities of laetrile were deemphasized; no physician, biochemist, or pharmacologist was even invited to speak. A sociologist commented on another presenter's critique, ". . . [Prof.] Rich's [critical] paper is the most difficult to treat because of the bias I perceive. . . . His view is as valid as mine, so I present these thoughts as an alternative view to consider. . . . Any analysis of laetrile must carry some bias; even neutrality is a bias. . . . [A]ny bias will do as well as another. . . . He should consider the degree to which his perceptions and conclusions depend on his particular bias rather than on 'objective fact'. . . ."

I received much the same treatment in 1976 from the sociology department at a major university when I presented the cultlike characteristics of the laetrile community and asked for help in investigating it. The sociologists felt there was little difference between the society of medical scientists and the society of laetrile advocates.

Through the nonjudgmental, relativist eyes of the medical sociologist, even fradulent medical schemes and cults are viewed as merely cultural differences. Observers' educated opinions become biases, whether they describe violation of laws of physics, chemistry, and pharmacology, or laws of the land.

POSTMODERNISM

The derivative of this relativism is the postmodern view exemplified by Michel Foucault, Jacques Derrida, Sandra Harding, Paul Feyerabend, and philosophers of science. They view science and knowledge as merely social constructions, relative to the individual's view, or to the society in which the knowledge is created.

Some versions of postmodernism deny the existence of an outside world or universe (or disease or treatment) that can be measured objectively and upon which one can take reasoned action. The result of this position is the dissolution of measurement—a world devoid of facts and judgment. Much of the liberal-arts and social-science academic community has been devoted to this view for several decades. Two generations of students have been educated in it, taking places in the legal community as attorneys and judges, politicians and officeholders, and in the media as reporters, editors, and producers. Administrators of granting agencies—both public and private—grounded in relativistic/constructivist principles, determine where and to whom research grants go. Prior to applying for an NIH grant to study the effects of traditional medical practices on chemotherapy compliance, I was told by a staffer to omit the word "compliance" if I wanted to he funded.

Editors and staffs of professional journals are affected by the "niceness" straightjacket. Courses in "CAM" are taught in most medical schools without critique or evaluation of validity. "Therapeutic Touch" is not just tolerated, but taught in nursing schools.

MONEY

There has always been a fringe of healers, doctor wannabes, willing to dispense information for a price, or just for the self-satisfaction of appearing to be real scientists and physicians. Their seeming reason for existence is to supply methods rejected by scientific biomedicine. Others make and sell products with debatable or no effects, competing with effective pharmaceuticals. All have succeeded in winning over a minority of the public that now has firm belief in the power of supplements, antioxidants, athletic fuel, brain food, and special diets. Bookstore sales on health, nutrition, and medicine are high, and magazine racks overflow. The competition for space is fierce. There has always been good grazing along the fringes of medicine.

But now wannabes are taking shark bites out of medicine's flesh. They have perfected techniques of sales, propaganda, legal maneuvering, and political contributing and have reached significant levels of influence. The supplement industry, of course, influenced Rep. Bill Richardson and Sen. Orrin Hatch, who wrote the Dietary Supplement Health and Education Act of 1994. The bill liberalized marketing of supplements and removed the Food and Drug Administration's preemptive control over unsafe products. Companies now market products without proof of effectiveness and flood the marketplace with unstandardized, sometimes toxic, herbs and supplements.

Organized chiropractic and other occupational guilds repeatedly seek increased scope of practice, claiming to be able to diagnose and treat as physicians. Political contributions from fringe practitioner guilds regularly retool legislatures.

Private foundations fund many "AM" activities and may be the largest source of "AM" funding. The $300-million Fetzer Foundation funded the Bill Moyers PBS TV series *Cancer and the Mind* and the 1993 Eisenberg *New England Journal of Medicine* "AM" study. It still funds the Beth Israel/Harvard and other medical school courses, postgraduate physician education courses, departments, and research projects. The Laing Foundation (>$1 million) funded the University of Maryland acupuncture (pain) program and other activities. The Rosenthal Foundation funds Columbia University's "AM" program to at least $750,000. The Templeton Foundation gives annual awards, funds research, and supports other nonprofit organizations for millions of dollars for support of spirituality and religion in medicine. Ten million dollars went to the University of California this year from the Osher Foundation for an "altmed" service. Endowments are in the hundreds of millions of dollars, with annual funding exceeding the $14-20 million per year of the Federal Office of Alternative Medicine.

These foundations are products of wealthy entrepreneurs with private ideologies they would like to see adopted by society. Financially strapped universities and medical schools accept these funds under conditions not acceptable a decade ago. A few years ago, Yale University declined a contribution from a conservative donor on ideological grounds, and was hailed by the academic community.

PROPAGANDA AND LANGUAGE DISTORTION

We now see a new use of an ancient tool used by experts at manipulation of the public mind. Even the words "holistic," "alternative," "complementary," "unconventional," and "unorthodox" are invented euphemisms intended to mislead. They are benign terms covering a vast array of practices—most of them unproved, dubious, disproved, absurd, and fraudulent. Any politician knows one must find an enemy, even a straw one, to win elections. The term, "slash, burn, and poison" was invented by laetrile advocates to demean ethical cancer medicine, and it worked and it stuck.

In a strange twist of the braid, constructivist sociologist-historians of medicine in an "alternative medicine" journal have already turned the tables on our analysis of language distortion and accused rationalist scientists' use of realistic terms like quackery, misrepresentation, and fraud of being merely prejudicial and biased. They call for more neutral terms to describe absurd methods like homeopathy. Thus the strings of constructivism and propaganda complement each other in the braid.

MISREPRESENTATION OF RESEARCH RESULTS

In the course of a legal action, I had opportunity to review the major papers claimed to be positive by homeopaths. We presented some analyses of these papers at the AAAS in 1997, in *Skeptical Inquirer* (summer 1997), and in other journals. Most of the alleged positive reports showed serious defects including selected end points, analysis of aggregated data as if they were homogeneous, extraordinarily large confidence intervals with minimal significance, selected reporting of differences in recorded curves, miscalculations and misrecording of data, omissions of control and other objective data, and combining different dis, ease categories into meta-analyses. Why peer reviewers miss such errors is unexplained. To make matters worse, another meta-analysis appearing in the *Lancet* in the fill of 1997 recorded the results of homeopathy studies at face value, despite the papers' faults. The meta-analysis is now a reference for the claim that homeopathy cannot be entirely explained by placebo action.

Once inaccuracies in "CAM" are reported as fact in medical literature, they are there for posterity. Even Hillary Clinton has quoted the seriously defective Byrd study on intercessory prayer in the coronary care unit as evidence for spirituality's effectiveness.

BAD DOCTORING

Good doctors know who the other good doctors are. One of the darkest, most secret, and little-mentioned factors in the "AM" controversy is that "AM" advocates are not in the higher ranks of good doctors. Many or most are probably in the lowest ranks of quality.

Although this is dangerous ground because of lack of data, there is clearly something wrong with the judgment of physicians who hold closely to ideologically driven methods that lack validity. Many of them have been disciplined by medical boards. The public usually has little sense for the quality of physicians, and there is little evidence that publication of lists of "best doctors" alters patient behavior. Most of us want to have our physicians be top quality, but apparently the customers of aberrant practitioners have other agendas in mind.

THE PRESS

The press is the major vector for the spread of "CAM" through its uncritical reporting and misrepresentation. Several times a year in most newspapers, a novice reporter claiming skepticism consults an "alternative" practitioner, often an acupuncturist, and reports that some chronic aggravation improved. Not reported is the fact that controlled trials show the method is not effective. Nor does the article follow up on how often or how much the symptom recurs over the next year or five. These are facts most physicians must have and must divulge before obtaining informed consent for a procedure.

The July 3, 1998, *San Jose Mercury News* bore a small *Washington Post* article about rural China's 70 percent infestation rate by various parasites, most commonly worms, resulting in malnutrition, decreased intelligence, and general weakening of the workforce. The article was buried on page DD5. The previous week's acupuncture article was on page 1B, complete with half-page photo. This kind of editorial treatment is typical.

The press is also often scammed. In the August 16, 1998, issue of *Parade* magazine, there appeared an article about the marvels of acupuncture, including a smiling woman undergoing chest surgery with only ear acupuncture for anesthesia. The photo appeared to be a fake, as did the story (chest surgery without intubation and heart bypass or cooling?). Such scams or cons—or variants on them—are widespread, and the press frequently falls for them.

So where are acupuncture and moxibustion when we need them? The worm infestation above apparently does not respond to "AM." The failure of traditional Chinese medicine in China and its maximum 18 percent usage there is a testimonial to modern biomedicine's success. But this is assumed not to interest the public; at least it seems not to interest the press.

The typical "AM" article highlights a few advocates, but presents the scientific view in two paragraphs—usually in the middle or toward the end of the article. (In television, the skeptical or scientific view is reduced to one or two 15-second bites. The pseudoscience view usually gets the last word.) This is called balanced reporting.

Reporters say, "My duty is to inform, to present both sides, and let the (readers, patients, etc.) make up their own minds." Although the material is often false or misrepresented, reporters (like some sociologists) seem to be answering to a higher calling. It is a presumptuous rationalization to avoid a major social responsibility.

POWER POLITICS

Traditionally, a distinguishing feature of quacks has been this: If they cannot prove their claims scientifically, they use the popular press and lobby for special privilege in legislatures. Twenty-seven states legalized laetrile in the 1970s and 1980s. Seven states have passed "access to medical treatment" (AMT) bills. These allow any licensed practitioner to practice any method within the legal scope of practice—proved or not—on any patient, provided "informed consent" is obtained. Regulatory boards, organized medicine, and public-service agencies oppose such bills. (Even now the Texas board is considering liberalizing regulations on aberrant practices to conform to policies resembling AMT bills.)

Pressure groups from the "CAM" community support these policies and contribute funds toward their passage. The primary pressure for

AMTs comes from "chelation therapy" physicians. (Chelation is a worthless "alternative" therapy for heart and vascular disease.) Political pressures, not public need or scientific validity, were behind the rise of chiropractic, acupuncture, and other methods.

One quick test for the usefulness of an "alternative" therapy is to ask oneself, what would happen if this therapy were tomorrow no longer available? How much would acupuncture and homeopathy be missed? How about antineoplastons, immunoaugmentive therapy, laetrile, and unsupervised megavitamins? If the public had never heard of them, the common health would not suffer a bit. On the other hand, how would the public handle absence of antibiotics, X-rays, anesthesia, and major operations?

GULLIBILITY, MISPERCEPTIONS, AND THE WILL TO BELIEVE

Much is written about these human traits, maybe too much to describe usefully here. So we recommend the reading of several books and critical research papers. Try *How We Know What Isn't So* by Thomas Gilovich, *The Psychology of Anomalous Experience* by Graham Reed, *How to Think about Weird Things* by Theodore Schick Jr. and Lewis Vaughn, any number of papers on belief perseverance by Lee Ross and others, *Cults in Our Midst* by Margaret Singer, *The Psychology of Transcendence* by Andrew Neher, *Deception and Self-Deception* by Richard Wiseman, "Memory" and "Eyewitness Testimony" by Elizabeth Loftus, and chapters by James Alcock and Barry Beyerstein in *The Encyclopedia of the Paranormal*. Throw in a few by Martin Gardner and James Randi for entertaining explorations of other oddities such as faith healers.

So the braid of the "AM" movement is complex and strong and will always lurk in our backgrounds, even if all human misery and disease were to be conquered. For now it grows into the interstices of scientific and ethical medicine's weaknesses and is fertilized by imagined faults. The movement has advanced socially and politically.

According to Prof. Edzard Ernst of Exeter University, the fascination with "AM" has peaked in the United Kingdom, and classes are poorly attended. The European Community is about to consider removing many worthless "AM" methods from lists for reimbursement. The same disenchantment may occur here in a few years. Yet we can learn from AM's existence and social successes. We can study misinterpretation of events and the formation of beliefs, increase our understanding of social movements, and perhaps tease out small kernels of benefits—even if only psychological—in some methods.

The challenge here is for us to increase our abilities to observe, measure, record, analyze, and reason, and not to allow the holes in our reality-sieve widen until we have lost our grip on it.

3

SCIENCE, POLITICS, AND ALTERNATIVE MEDICINE
What Physicians Should Know

Saul Green, Ph.D.

THE PHRASE ALTERNATIVE MEDICINE (AM) ENCOMPASSES A BROAD SPECtrum of treatments whose rationale and clinical effectiveness have never been proven but which are nevertheless recommended by their practitioners for use instead of scientifically established medical treatments.[1,2,3] Although the creators of these nostrums claim their effectiveness is based on good science, their publications show their only support to be unverifiable patient anecdotes.[4] The fact that AM practitioners willingly offer anecdotes as "proofs" betrays their ignorance of the fact that it is the scientific process that generates clinically significant data. Since no one characteristic signals the presence of fraud in AM, all potential users of these treatments must question the validity and the veracity of all the claims made for these treatments by objectively reading the descriptions of them that are found in books and magazines which are sold in bookstores, supermarkets, and at newspaper kiosks.

AM is practiced in one of two ways. In the first, actual substances are used which are said to activate existing body functions which then fight the disease naturally.[3] These substances may be in special diets, in coffee enemas, in Chinese herbs, in vitamins, in apricot pits (Laetrile). They may be concoctions prepared by the practitioner such as the camphor in 714-X, components from human urine (antineoplastons), pills containing hydrogen peroxide, hydrazine sulfate, or selenium soaps or gaseous ozone.

33

In the second way, tangible chemical substances are not involved. Instead, mystical rites are used to "call up" the patients' inate "healing powers." These rituals include tai chi, ayurveda, shiatsu, chakra healing, qigong therapy, acupuncture, visualization, meditation, faith healing, kirlian analysis, numerology, kinesiology, aroma therapy, and therapeutic touch.[5] As there is no objective rationale offered for the mechanism by which these rituals affect the disease process, they are untestable. Clearly, the patients willingness to submit to them is due entirely to their blind faith in the practitioner.[3]

AM practitioners treat patients according to the particular system they favor, not according to the distinct clinical condition of the patient. It is clear that the rationales they give for these treatments are not based on evidence from controlled clinical research trials but on concepts the healer knows the patient wants to believe in. At this point the reader may ask, " If it is easy to detect the fraud in AM treatments, why do so many patients choose to use them?" Some of the reasons may be that:

- Cures for many diseases do not exist and responsible medical scientists will not offer patients the (false) hope of medical miracles.
- Reporters prefer to write about the miracle cures claimed by AM practitioners because reporting the facts about cancer does not sell copy.
- Patients feel empathy for AM practitioners who allege they are "victims" of a greedy establishment and oppressive goverment regulatory agencies.
- The language used by AM proponents has converted what was once a clearly understood and simple dichotomy—quackery vs. conventional medicine—into a continuum of phrases that conveys a message of "hope." For example: "organic" suggests that a product grown using only natural fertilizer (manure) is more healthful; "natural" suggests that a product synthesized by metabolic processes of plants or animals must be safe; "healing" suggests activation of inate, spiritual "repair" processes that the patient alone controls.

AM therapists say that many of the treatments they offer are based on "ancient wisdom."[6] Thus they use laxatives and coffee enemas to purge the body of noxious humors or they practice mystic rituals to exhort the mind to cause "the patients body" to destroy tumors. More modern AMers use injections of live embryonic sheep cells to prevent aging. They infuse EDTA to "clean the calcium out of atherosclerotic plaque," gaseous ozone to reoxygenate "anaerobic" cancer tissues or kill the AIDS virus or urinary waste products to "normalize" cancer cells. Some direct patients to swallow capsules containing beef pancreatic enzymes to digest tumors, hydrazine sulphate to reverse tumor glycolysis, raw Chinese herbs to prevent cancer, megadoses of vitamin C to reverse harmful oxidative processes, and shark cartilage to block tumor angiogenesis. Homeopaths sell the "water" from which the "active substance" has been totally removed by serial dilution, saying that violent shaking of the solution between dilutions (succusion) potentizes the water and causes it to remember the medicine that was once in it.[7]

Diseases like cancer are not easily detectable in their early stages. When symptoms appear and diagnosis is possible, the available treatments may be painful, disabling, or mutilating. They will most certainly be costly. Sadly there are no guaranteed cures. If the patient endures the toxicity of chemotherapy, or the disfigurement of surgery and radiation and the treatment fails, then he or she and their family are left with the terrible anxiety attendant to the continued presence and possible progression of the disease. In such circumstances, the patients' search for "hope" is driven by desperation and they become fair game for those who willingly and glibly offer natural, safe remedies that *may* result in *healing*. In this frame of mind, a high level of intelligence doesn't guarantee that the patient will recognize the false hope present in the word "healing." The distraught patient wants so desperately to be saved that healing becomes synonymous with curing.

AM practitioners don't mean "cure" when they say "heal." In his book, *Choices in Healing*,[8] Michael Lerner defines a cure as the treatment that removes all medical evidence of the disease and allows the patient to live as long as he would have lived had he never become ill. Healing he says is an inner process which takes place at many levels including the psychological and the spiritual. In healing the patient moves toward God, makes a deeper connection with nature and achieves inner peace. Author Burton Goldberg[9] describes healing as the internal process of "becoming whole," the establishment of a harmonious relationship with ones' social and familial sphere, indeed with ones entire environment. Thus it pertains to all levels of a persons being and *the most powerful alternative cancer therapies* are those aimed at strengthening all these levels at the same time. They do this by reducing the body's *toxic* burden while enhancing its multifaceted self-healing capacities and bringing the true character of the individual into focus and healthy expression.

These statements may cause a patient to think he is hearing about a cure, but in fact they say nothing about stopping or reversing the disease process. To truly understand what they are being told, patients considering an AM treatment should demand to know: What are the self-healing (anticancer) capacities of my body; How were they identified and by whom; Which "toxic burdens" caused the cancer in my body; Will the healing your describe make my tumor to go away? Patients must ask themselves, "Am I going to a doctor to become whole, to achieve a harmonious relationship with my social and familial environment and to become one with the universe, or *am I going to be cured?*" Most especially they should ask the AM practitioner, "If healing is a highly personal "inner" process, is it my fault when the treatment fails?"

The AM practitioner recruits followers by assuming various guises.

As the "concerned citizen" he appeals to wealthy and prominent citizens who mistrust the medical establishment or have a vested interests in the products he is using. They use their social and political influence to lobby goverment officials, they fund television "specials," they publish "Newsletters" advertising his treatment. "Believers" in Congress introduce and influence passage legislation to keep agencies like FDA from regulating manufacture and sale of the health food supplements used in AM (i.e., Senate Bill S.2140, passed in 1994 through efforts of Sens. Harkin and Hatch.) Those who object to the practice of AM are characterized as being anti-God and un-American because they want to block the patients " Freedom of Choice."

As the "healer" he assumes the image of the God-fearing, caring physician who has no interest in money. He uses his "healed" patients to defend his claims by having them read from his prepared script. In doing this, they are deaf to questions about his lack of credentials, his flawed science and the absence of all clinical evidence that his treatment is effective. They charge that their "regular" doctors offered them no hope but still prescribed the "cutting, burning or poisoning" of orthodox medicine. They insist that the establishment doctors were proven wrong when their beloved healers treatments "saved" them.

As the "scientist" he poses as the dedicated researcher who claims success because he understands the ancient healing arts as well as the latest facts of modern medical science. When his claims are rebutted by highly respected scientific authorities, he assures his flock that, like all great scientists in the past, his concepts are so advanced, they can't be understood by establishment doctors and that is why they are repudiated.

AM practitioners know that a short-lived clinical improvement doesn't mean the treatment works, that anecdotes aren't evidence of a cure and that even a promise of "healing" will cheer up patients, improve their appetites and alter their perception of pain. They know that such responses are not due to the AM treatment but are "placebo" effects.[10] The word *placebo* comes from the Latin, meaning "I will please." It is not an AM treatment. In the basic research lab a placebo is the base line from which the investigator measures the activity of the substance he is studying. When the word placebo is used clinically it refers to specific effects that are generated in the patient by the patient-doctor relationship. This placebo effect is strictly limited to perceptual phenomena like symptoms and pain. It does not cause the repair of damaged tissue or alter the progress of a disease. It seems clear therefore, that an awareness of these facts coupled with the patients eagerness to pay huge sums for "hope" is what makes the practice of AM such an enormously successful business.

Every medical scientist lives with the challenge," PROVE IT!" In the basic research laboratory, they strive to produce experimental evidence which will support their hypothesis and which can be independently confirmed by others. Confirmation that the research results support a conclusion of significant medical value occurs only after all facets of the work are peer reviewed and accepted for publication in a reputable scientific journal. It is not the academic stature, the "common sense" of the theory, the preeminence of political supporters, or the illusions of patients that make the researchers conclusions valid. It is whether the experimental results can be replicated and validated by independent investigators.

In clinical research the investigator works to determine if the substances which showed promise in the preclinical research are safe and effective for general medical use in humans. For this, the U.S. Food and Drug Administration (FDA) has developed guidelines for the clinical evaluation of a new drug. These present the clinical researcher with recommended approaches to the study of new drugs in man. They are: Screening—drug testing in animals to determine their potential for use against human cancer. Toxicology—determination of how a drug is handled by the tissues of experimental animal. Phase I—determination of the safety of the new drug in healthy volunteers to determine its chemical actions in the body, how it is absorbed, how it should be administered, the safe dosage levels and how well it is tolerated. Phase II—determination of the efficacy of the drug in patients who have specific diseases using the dosages proven to be safe in Phase I. Phase III—comparison of the effectiveness of the experimental with that of existing standard therapy, in a large number of subjects with defined disease. when analyzed in conjunction with the council of outstanding experts in the field, the results of these clinical trials represent acceptable conclusions about the safety and efficacy of the new drug which will allow for its integration into a primary treatment program perhaps in combination with surgery and or radiation.

The elements that make up a good clinical trial include rigorous control and objective interpretation of data based on an intimate knowledge of the biology of normal tissue, the cause of the disease and the biochemical changes that occur as the disease progresses. The medical researcher who is testing the therapy must learn all he can about the chemical composition, specificity, metabolism, toxicity and excretion rates of each of the treatment substances so the patients clinical progress can be accurately monitored. Finally each patient must be closely followed for a significant period of time after the treatment ends, so all after effects can be noted. Only when these criteria are met can a valid conclusion be reached about the efficacy of a new treatment. Accordingly, every physician who has a patient that is considering an AM treatment, must ask that patient, "Has the treatment the AM person is offering you ever been tested for safety and effectiveness by a process like the one required by FDA as described above?"

No one should be surprised to learn that government agencies respond to pressure from Congress and that Congressmen are lobbied by vested interest groups from their states. When the Congressmen are already "confirmed believers" in a cause, the pressure they can exert becomes intense. It was just such pressure that caused the office of Technology Assessment (OTA) of the NIH to hold extensive hearings on the subject of AM treatments in 1989. Almost without exception those who were invited to present talks were AM practitioners or their proponents and each one of them strongly affirmed the *right* of each of the others to practice their own brand of therapy. This was followed by descriptions of the "unbelievable" healings that individual treatments were said to have produced. Of interest was the fact that not one of the presenting practitioners had personally tested the safety or efficacy of the AM treatment of another nor did they recommend use of any but their own. In September of 1990 the OTA, on advice from its board of scientific advisors, concluded that they could not endorse the use of any AM treatment.[2]

In the years before 1992, Senator Tom Harkin's friend, "true believer" Berkeley Bedell (Representative-Iowa) was spreading the word of miracle AM cures.[12] Bedell proclaimed that his prostate cancer, which had already been successfully treated with conventional medicine, was uncured. Accordingly, he sought out Gaston Naesens, a Canadian "healer" with two convictions for illegally practicing medicine in Europe. Naessons advertised that he had a cure for prostate cancer. After allowing Naessens to inject him with 714-X, a mixture of camphor, mineral salts, alcohol and water, Bedell declared himself cured.[12] Another example of Bedells willingness to "believe" was revealed when he announced that he cured his Lyme disease by buying and drinking the first milk (colostrum) secreted by the mammary glands of a Lyme infected cow. When the Minnesota farmer who owned the cow was arrested for practicing medicine without a license, Bedell paid his legal fees and testified in his behalf.[13]

Senator Harkin became a full-fledged "true believer" after Bedell introduced him to Royden Brown, the owner of a company that manufactured Bee Pollen capsules. Brown told Harkin that Bee Pollen would cure all his allergies so Harkin swallowed 250 capsules over five days. He then publicly declared that all his allergies had been cured.[12] In 1992, Harkin was chairman of the Senate Appropriations subcommittee in charge of NIH funding. Using the power of this office and under the influence of the group of "healers" he had collected around himself, Harkin fathered the office of Alternative Medicine (OAM). At OAM's birth, Harkin announced it would work to weed the quackery out of AM.[14] Considering the fact that most of the members of OAM's first advisory council were either AM practitioners or proponents, his mandate to them could well have been, "Do whatever is necessary to get AM into mainstream medicine." Notwithstanding the fact that OAMS first annual budget was only 2 million dollars per year, they quickly gave away about half of it for studies on the clinical effectiveness of prayer, aroma therapy, therapeutic touch, homeopathy and mind-body healing.[15] Seven years have now passed and the OAM budget has risen to 20 million dollars. Although new grants continue to be doled out, no results confirming the effectiveness of AM have been published in reputable peer reviewed medical journals and not one AM treatment has been labeled "quackery."

As a result of the media coverage of AM miracle cures, some independent clinical researchers tested the claims being made. Using double blindedplacebo controlled trials, the treatments tested and reported on in peer-reviewed journals were: laetrile,[16] acupuncture,[17] chelation,[18] hydrazine sulfate,[19] and vitamin C.[20] The results demonstrated that these treatments were clinically worthless. Of course, these results were refuted by AM proponents who charged, as they always did, that the test substances were administered incorrectly, the dosages used were too high, too low, or were adulterated, that drugs were given to inhibit or inactivate the treatment and that the clinical data was improperly collected and incorrectly analyzed. This, they said, proves that the medical, pharmaceutical, and insurance establishments are engaged in a continuing conspiracy to keep "safe, effective and inexpensive" new treatments from reaching the public.

Just what can an objective review of the published literature of an alternative medicine practitioner reveal? A brief answer is found in a paper published in JAMA in June of 1992 (22). The subject was the claim by Stanislaw R. Burzynski, M.D., that he discovered anticancer peptides in human urine while doing research in medical school. He named them antineoplastons. A critical examination of the claims made in Dr. Burzynski's own publications showed: that none of the papers he co-authored while in medical school (1964–1970), mentioned research in human cancer, antineoplastons or urine; that his advanced degree was the

DMSc not the Ph.D.; that none of the peptides he worked with were ever shown to be able to "normalize" human cancer cells; that within one year of announcing his theory of antineoplastons, he treated 21 cancer patients with antineoplaton A, a urine fraction for which no safety or efficacy testing had been done; that the five antineoplastons he produced from antineoplaston A, appeared to be all the same; that antineoplaston A-10 which he produced from fraction A-2, was an insoluble product, formed from phenylacetylglutamine (PAG) a substance normally present in human urine; that when PAG is acidified and concentrated A-10 is formed; that insoluble A-10 is not solubilized by treatment with NaOH but is hydrolyzed back to the original PAG; that PAG has little or no activity against cancer cells in culture; that the "soluble" A-10 currently being used as a treatment for human cancer is PAG.

People are usually outraged when they learn they have been "conned." For some reason, patients and their families do not feel victimized after learning they have spent huge sums on worthless AM treatments. Perhaps they are embarrassed by their gullibility or they rationalize the cost as "gratitude" for the brief respite from terror that their purchase of "false hope" brought to a loved one. This state of mind was described by Oliver Wendell Holmes in 1891.[21] He wrote:

> There is nothing that men will not do to recover their health and save their lives. They have submitted to being half drowned in water, choked with gases, buried to their chins in earth, seared with hot irons, crimped with knives, had needles thrust into their flesh, had fires kindled on their skin, and swallowed all sorts of abominations. Then they pay for all this as if scalding were a privilege, blisters a blessing and leeches a luxury. What more can be asked for as proof of their sincerity?

The knowing sale of false hope to a terrified cancer patient has got to be one of the lowest forms of human behavior. To counter it, healthcare professionals must make a concerted effort to learn as much as possible about these treatments and their purveyors. In that way they can act as knowledgeable sources of rational information for those patients who wish to exercise their right to Freedom of Informed Choice. With truth at their disposal, patients can tell when they are getting the very best possible care from a responsible physician who understands their needs and is honestly and knowledgeably working to solve their clinical problems.

The author is indebted to Sylvia A. Karchmar for editing the manuscript and offering suggestions for making it "user" friendly.

NOTES

(**Denotes Uncritical Advocacy)

1. Barrett, S. and Jarvis, Wm. T. (eds). *The Health Robbers: A Close Look At Quackery in America.* Amherst, N.Y. Prometheus Books. 1993

2. Unconventional Cancer Treatments. Office of Technology Assessment. OTA-H405, Washington D.C., U.S. Government Printing Office. 1990

3. Cassileth, BR. *The Alternative Medical Handbook.* New York, London. W.W. Norton and Co. 1998.

4. **Alternative Medicine-Expanding Medical Horizons. Prepared under the auspices of the Workshop on Alternative Medicine. Chantilly, VA. 1992

5. Raso, J. *The Dictionary of Metaphysical Healthcare: Alternative Medicine, Paranormal Healing and Related Methods.* Loma Linda, CA. The National Council Against Health Fraud. 1996

6. Cramp, AJ. Nostrums, *Quackery and Allied Matters Affecting the Public Health.* Vol II, Chicago Ill., AMA Press, 1921.

7. **Cummings S. and Ullman D. *Homeopathic Medicines.* Los Angeles, CA. JP Tarcher Inc. 1991

8. ***Choices in Healing.* Michael Lerner, PhD. The MIT Press, Cambridge Mass. and London, England. 1994.

9. **Diamond JW, Cowden WL, with Goldberg, B. Alternative medicine-Definitive Future Medicine Publishing Inc. Tiburon, CA. 1997

10. Shapiro, AK, and Shapiro, E. *The Powerful Placebo: From Ancient Priest to Modern Physician.* Baltimore, Johns Hopkins University Press, 1997.

11. Crout JR, Finkel MJ. Guidelines for the Clinical Evaluation of Antineoplastic Drugs. Food and Drug Administration, HHS,81-3112. 1981.

12. Budianski, S., Cures or "quackery." How Senator Harkin shaped federal research on alternative medicine. *U.S. News & World Report.* pp. 48–51. July, 1995.

13. Minnesota Milk Cure Case. *Minneapolis Star Tribune*. March 16, 1995

14. Angier, N. U.S. Opens the Door Just a Crack to Alternative Medicine. *New York Times*, Sunday, January 10, 1993.

15. Stern, M. Chief, NIH News. NIH, Office of Alternative Medicine, Grant Recipients. To investigate and validate alternative medical practices. Fiscal Year, 1993.

16. Moertel CG, et al. A clinical trial of Amygdalin (laetrile) in the treatment of human cancer. *N. Engl J Med* 306:201-206: 1982

17. Sampson, W. et al, Acupuncture- A position paper of the National Council Against Health Fraud. *Clinical Journal of Pain*. 7:162-166:1991

18. Ernst E, Chelation therapy for peripheral arterial occlusive disease; A systematic review. *Circulation*. 96:1031-1033:1997

19. Chlebowski RT, et al. Hydrazine sulfate in cancer patients with weight loss. A placebo controlled clinical experience. *Cancer* 59: 406-410: 1987

20. Moertel CG et al. High dose vitamin C versus placebo in the treatment of patients with advanced cancer who had no prior chemotherapy. A randomized double blind comparison. *N Engl J Med* 312: 137-142:1985

21. Holmes OW. *Medical Essays*. Boston: Houghton Miffin. 1891.

22. Green, S. Antineoplastons—An Unproved Cancer Therapy. *JAMA*, 267:#21: 29242928: 1992.

PSYCHOLOGY
AND
BELIEF

4

ALTERNATIVE MEDICINE AND THE PSYCHOLOGY OF BELIEF

James E. Alcock

IN 1988, I WAS PART OF A SIX-PERSON DELEGATION FROM THE COMMITTEE for the Scientific Investigation of Claims of the Paranormal (CSICOP) that visited the People's Republic of China. We had been invited to investigate (i) Qi Gong, a vitalistic belief system that, among other things, is employed to diagnose and heal disease, and (ii) the abilities of a group of children who, it was claimed, could read with their armpits. During our stay in Beijing, I developed a very sore throat, due, I thought, to the visibly polluted air. This made it difficult to engage in conversations and deliver the speeches that were expected of us. Eventually, I was taken to the outpatient clinic at Beijing Hospital, and after a very brief examination, was given two medications. The first, labelled in both Chinese and English, was erythromycin, an antibiotic. That seemed reasonable enough for what I thought to be a bronchial infection. The second medication bore the label Chuanbeiye, and the chief ingredients were listed as "snake bile, tendril-leafed fritillary bulb, and almond, etc." Our interpreter assured me that she always relied on the snake bile preparation whenever she had any throat problems, but despite her earnest testimonial, I declined to use it. I relied instead upon the erythromycin, and within a couple of days, my throat recovered. Offered folk medicine and snake oil, I had chosen scientific Western medicine and was healed by it.

Or so I thought. After our return from China, Paul Kurtz recounted this incident in an article in CSICOP's journal, the *Skeptical Inquirer*. A few months later, an *SI* reader, Dr. Raymond Cloutier, wrote:

> All too often bronchial infections are due to viruses and therefore not treatable with antibiotics. Unfortunately, there is such a demand from the lay public to treat everything with antibiotics that it is not unusual for the encumbered physician to prescribe them for infections they know cannot be helped by antibiotics.

Dr. Cloutier concluded with this irony:

> If this was a viral infection, then the antibiotic and the snake bile were of equal efficacy.

But I got better, didn't I? Doesn't that tell me that the antibiotic worked?

When we talk about the appeal of this treatment or that treatment, this is what is at the heart of it all—we use medicines because they seem to work. If we get better, we naturally credit the treatment (whether it had any effect or not). And when we do not improve, we naturally assume that the treatment did not work, and we may then seek out other therapies that might.

So-called alternative or complementary therapies are popular only to the extent that they can satisfy some people's needs better than conventional medical therapies do. If every visit to the family physician cured our complaints and satisfied our needs (the two are not necessarily the same), then the vast majority of people would never consider alternate therapies. And if, once people tried alternative therapies, they did not seem to be effective, most people would stop using them and they would eventually die out.

It is a mistake to assume that people who use unproven or even disproven therapies are necessarily less rational, less sensible, or even less educated than those who do not. (Most surveys show that, on average, users of alternative medicine tend to have more years of formal education than nonusers—a by-product of the fact that these users must generally pay out of their own pockets and thus must have more disposable income.)[1] No one that I have ever met would knowingly submit to treatment that he or she believed to be totally useless or harmful. We pursue a therapy because we believe, or at least hope, that it may work. (This does not refer, of course, to the radical fringe, people for whom use of alternative medicine is an integral part of an overarching sociopolitical, antiscience, or New Age worldview.)

The interesting question is how we come to believe that a therapy may be worthwhile. And since none of us is likely (even if we possess the necessary knowledge, skills, and wherewithal) to carry out clinical trials before choosing a treatment for the first time, we will ultimately base our initial decision on our faith in others' opinions and even, perhaps, others' research. However, once we decide to try a therapy, our own experience becomes very important, and a variety of psychological factors come into play that may help persuade us that the therapy is effective, even if it is not.

Most people turn to and believe in alternative therapies for the same reasons they turn to and believe in evidence-based medicine. Most users of alternative medicine are ignorant of, and uninterested in, the theoretical basis of homeopathy or chiropractic or naturopathy, just as most users of evidence-based medicine are ignorant of and uninterested in its theoretical underpinnings. Physicians have taught us not to enquire too much about what is in this tablet or how that injection works. We wouldn't be able to understand it anyway, and after all, we have come to the physician because we trust that he or she understands so that we don't have to. Most people who keep using alternative therapies do so because they believe it helps, just as is the case with those who continue to go back for treatment with evidence-based therapies.

In the end, it boils down to what our individual belief systems incline us to accept as evidence. In this article, I shall discuss how we learn about causality, how our beliefs and our trust develop, and how this shapes our concepts of illness and healing. It is through these mechanisms that people come to have confidence in any therapy, evidence-based or not, and effective or not.

HOW WE LEARN ABOUT CAUSALITY

When I stated earlier that the antibiotic made me better, what did that statement actually mean? In reality, all that happened was that two events occurred in succession: One, I took the medicine, and two, not too long afterward, I felt better. Yet, my conclusion was a causal one: The medicine made me better. That is consistent with my limited knowledge of medicine and my expectations. Since I knew nothing directly about the causal link, or even for sure if there was one, my judgment was really magical thinking. Magical thinking describes what happens when we experience two successive events and conclude that the first event caused the second, without any concern for the putative causal link. All humans are to some degree magical thinkers. Until recently, most psychologists used to think that textbook logic and reasoning practices were the "default mode," and that when people engaged in magical or superstitious thinking it was some kind of pathology, a deviation from the inbred norm. Research has taught us, however, that magical thinking (i.e., "quick-and-dirty" reasoning tactics that get it more or less right a sufficient portion of the time to be useful) is our first line of attack when reckoning with the world—logical, analytical reasoning is a fragile add-on that must be painstakingly learned.[2,3,4]

We actually have two quite distinct information-processing systems in our brains and nervous systems that lead us to conclusions about causality. On the one hand, we learn quickly from direct experience. Put your finger in a live lamp socket, and your experience quickly teaches you not to do that again. This is experiential learning. No knowledge of electricity, no understanding of physics, is necessary. A dumb animal would learn as quickly not to touch the socket again. On the other hand, we also process information in an intellectual manner, through reasoning, logic, and analysis. Through intellectual learning, we come to know that a flow of electrons races down our finger when we touch a live contact point in the socket, and we can learn to avoid touching sockets even if we have never had any direct experience with them.

Experiential learning. Experiential learning occurs at a primitive level—it is automatic, rapid, and often tied up with emotional reactions.

It requires no formal teaching, no practice, no theoretical understanding, no contemplation, no logic. It is based on patterns that we detect in the world around us.

We enter this world superbly equipped to learn quickly about our environment. Our nervous systems are bombarded with an unending shower of sensory stimulation from both within and without our bodies. We are able at birth to begin to find patterns in this stimulation, to make sense out of it. To do so we rely on two factors—temporal contiguity and stimulus generalization. By temporal contiguity, I mean that events that occur closely together in time have a special impact on our nervous systems; they set up an "association" in our brains. Touch a hot stove, feel pain, and the nervous system "learns" to avoid the hot stove. And then, by the process of stimulus generalization, one learns not only to avoid that stove, the one that caused the pain, but other stoves and any object that looks similar to that stove. In other words, without the need for any reasoning or logic or words or understanding, we quickly internalize some "knowledge" about the world—don't touch stoves; they cause pain. The importance of such learning for survival is obvious. Yet, again, note the imputation of causality, when all we really experience is temporal contiguity. This applies just as readily to positive outcomes: Take a pill and the headache goes away. We attribute the pain relief to the pill.

Asymmetric effect of pairing and nonpairing: It is important to understand, as I have discussed in detail elsewhere,[5,6] that we do not easily unlearn associations between important events. If the infant, by accident, touches the same stove a day later, but this time it is cold and so no pain occurs, his or her nervous system does not simply reset to itself to zero so far as stoves are concerned. Obviously, this would not be very adaptive in terms of our survival: The rabbit that encounters a snarling, biting fox and lives to remember it would not be well served by a nervous system that unlearns the fear of foxes, just because on one occasion, the rabbit encounters a fox that makes no effort to turn it into dinner. The association set up by the co-occurrence of two significant events is not easily undone. If your migraine went away last week when you took a pill, but did not abate when you took another pill today, would you decide that the pill does not work after all? Not likely.

Intermittent reinforcement: Indeed, what happens if, ten times in a row, the child accidentally brushes against the stove, but the stove is cool? With an accumulation of such experiences, the association between stove and pain will gradually weaken, but—and this is a very important "but"—if every now and then touching the stove produces pain, this results in an even more enduring association between stove and pain, for one automatically learns that the fact that the stove was harmless enough—even a number of times in a row—does not mean that it will not burn the next time. Occasional, intermittent reinforcement produces even more enduring associations than continuous reinforcement—if you doubt this fact, just watch the "one-armed bandit" players in any casino for a while. The intermittent reinforcement effect is just as true for the pill that is followed by relief every now and then, if there is no other apparent relief mechanism available.

Superstitious conditioning: I have been discussing a situation where there actually is a causal relationship between the hot stove and pain and perhaps between pill and relief. However, our nervous systems have no direct way of knowing that. That conclusion belongs to the realm of reason, not experience. Suppose that by happenstance, a child reaches for a new toy just as there is a terrible clap of thunder that frightens him or her. The association will be set up between toy and the fearful noise, and the child may from now on avoid that toy. This is referred to as superstitious conditioning. It is interesting to note that the term "superstitious" is applied by the observer who knows that there really is not a causal link. In fact, most of the time, when we are inferring causality, we cannot really tell whether there is a causal link or not. We take the vitamin C and feel better, or we don't catch a cold; did one cause the other? We are likely to think so—especially if we have other reasons—authority, testimonials, and beliefs consistent with that interpretation. Only very careful and time-consuming research can really tell us whether there is any causality involved at all.

Intellectual learning. Be that as it may, while our experiential learning is of vital importance for survival, the major reason that we have triumphed over other species and made them part of our food chain, rather than the other way around, is that we possess relatively advanced cognitive abilities. With our rich heritage of logical analysis and our culturally codified knowledge base, we are able, through contemplation, to estimate the value and meaning of most things around us. And through our highly efficacious communication abilities, we can teach our children about "how things work," without the need for them to go out and experience everything firsthand, or to develop intellectual understanding from basic principles. (Now, if we could only get them to pay attention!)

Yet, we have to learn how to learn in this way. We have to learn logic. We have to learn how to organize our knowledge into categories and categories into an explanatory framework. We have to learn that surface appearances don't always relate to underlying realities. And just as it took civilization thousands of years to develop what we think of today as logic and scientific inquiry, so each individual spends many years in formal education. In this way, each of us is taught how to think in a logical manner, although, strangely enough, not all that much of children's formal education is devoted to developing logical abilities that will serve them well in everyday life. There is no reason why we could not teach children in grade 5 about the need for double-blind randomized clinical trials, especially if we used age-appropriate, attention-grabbing examples. They could understand, and it would be a big step toward fostering critical thinkers, savvy consumers, and informed voters.

Human beings are constantly seeking to "understand." We want explanations for events around us. What was that noise in the garage? There should be no one in there—is it a raccoon, a burglar, the wind, or am I just "hearing things"? Why isn't my doctor curing my condition? We make causal attributions continually—the floor is wet because the shower curtain was not all the way into the bathtub. The tree branch was blown down by the wind. Martha ignored me because she is envious. Harry was nice to me because he wants to borrow some money. I got better because I took the erythromycin. And most of us are uncomfortable when we are unable to assign causes to events. "Harry is floating in midair. Shucks, that is strange; but I don't have an explanation, so I will just forget about it." Martha recovered from terminal cancer, when the doctors said she would die—it must have been the laetrile that saved her, or it must have been the prayer. Most of us, in our personal lives, have a hard time accepting ambiguity, accepting that sometimes we just don't know.

Conflicts between the experiential and the intellectual. As determined as we may be to base our decisions on fact, not faith; intellect, not emotion; reason, not rhetoric; we can do so only up to a point. Like it or not, our lives are to a considerable degree governed by primitive associations hardened into our nervous systems by experience.

There will be times where we "know" one thing intellectually, but "feel" strongly something else. You may "know" that the garter snake in the cage cannot really hurt you, but you cannot push yourself to touch it. You may "know" that flying through turbulence is not dangerous and no different than being on a motor boat on some choppy water, but nonetheless, you may feel irrational, even incapacitating, fear.

What do we do when faced with the choice between going with logic or emotion, reason or intuition? As much as we may be dedicated to reason, emotion has a very forceful way of making us an offer that is hard to refuse. As the public speaker seized by stage fright knows all too well, we cannot by virtue of rationality or willpower simply turn off those powerful feelings—and they are often impossible to ignore. Sometimes, the easiest way to reduce the conflict is to bring the intellect into line with the emotions, because most often we cannot do the opposite.[7] "Yes, airplanes are dangerous—my fear is justified." And if evidence-based medicine can't cure you, and alternative medicine says it can, which do you believe? Many people experience a decrease in anxiety if they accept the alternative healer's claims, and that anxiety relief may thwart whatever challenges are mounted by data and intellect.

BELIEFS

Our beliefs are, in essence, our expectations about the world around us. I believe the road continues on the other side of the hill. I believe that submitting to surgery will take away the pain in my belly, even it the pain initially increases. I believe that oil of tangerine will cure my headaches.

But where do our beliefs originate?

- From direct experience: I had a bad headache, took oil of tangerine and it went away.
- From watching others: Mum always took oil of tangerine whenever she had a headache.

- From logical, analytical thought—evaluating research on oil of tangerine.
- From authority, being taught directly by parents, teachers, media: "Now children, don't forget to take your oil of tangerine."

Authority is, of course, a primary source of belief. We spend many years in school, being pushed to master sets of facts provided by authority, most of which we have very limited means to challenge. Similarly, the media bombard us with assertions that many are inclined to accept because, "They couldn't say that on TV if it weren't true, could they?" And our most unshakeable beliefs are often those for which we have no direct experiential support, but have come down to us from one authority or another, and are shared by people around us. For example, we learn that the earth is not flat—despite whatever our direct experience of it might suggest, and even though it is the rare person indeed who has ever actually tried to conduct research into the claim. Most would not even know where to begin. But we do not hear many people expressing doubt on the matter. We all accepted what was, initially at least, handed down by authority. And if someone in authority, even if that authority is self-proclaimed, tells me to reduce the amount of fat in my diet in order to preserve my health, or tells me to take St. John's Wort if I am depressed, why shouldn't I believe?

Our beliefs become integrated into a fabric that makes them difficult to change, even if information that contradicts them comes along.[8] If I come to believe that chiropractic is effective therapy, then even if research studies find no benefit, "it must work—it helped my back, my uncle swears by it, health insurance covers it, a regulatory body supervises it. One study isn't going to convince me that all those people are wrong." This is as true for our personal beliefs about aspirin or penicillin as it is for chiropractic or Echinacea.

Of course, the social support resulting from a sharing of belief is important. If you have never heard of oil of tangerine until I mention it, you may hesitate to take it, but if you have read testimonials about its virtues; if you have other acquaintances who use it, it is more likely that you will try it, and you will want it to work. You may reason, "What's the harm—if it doesn't work, at least it can't hurt me"—or so many people are predisposed to believe about alternative therapies.

Of course, we do learn to be skeptical, too. We soon learn that not all sources of information are equally reliable, and as we become better educated by life, we come to accept information from some sources almost without question, while routinely discrediting information from other sources. But how do we choose our sources, our authorities? I allow certain people wearing white coats to inject substances into my veins, almost at their whim, or to put their fingers in orifices that they were not designed to enter, without being told anything other than the potion or the prodding will have a therapeutic or diagnostic benefit. Yet, certain other people in white coats who may want to give my neck a good twist or insert tiny needles into my skin with the promise of bringing benefit I do not allow near me. Why not? We all have learned to choose our authorities.

ILLNESS AND HEALING

I want now to turn to a series of questions about illness and healing:

How do we know we are ill?

Language is a wonderful tool for disseminating knowledge about most things in our world. However, since we have no method of determining whether or not a child is in pain, or whether or not a child is frightened or worried, except by judging his or her behavior, how do we know what a child is feeling? Of course, we do not, not before the child can talk. We may measure the child's temperature and decide that there is fever, but is the inference that the child feels in pain or sickly necessarily correct? We don't know.

We teach young children about their emotional states, about pain, about sickness, by our judgments of what they must be feeling or should be feeling. We teach them the language of pain and illness: "I feel like I am going to die" or, "It's nothing, just a flesh wound." We teach children to relax or to worry, based on our reactions to our definition of what is going on inside them. We teach children—and this is in part culturally based of course, a sick role—how they are to react—to be passive, dependent, let the parent or doctor take care of them.[9] And since, even as we grow up, the innards of our bodies remain to a very large extent unknown to us, we teach children to rely for the most part on other people—on authorities—to tell them what is wrong and to fix the problem. We learn that when we are sick, our job as patient is to follow orders and the doctor's job is to make us better.

But I come back to the question of how we know we are sick. Generally, it is simply because we don't feel well, or we are vomiting, or we are always tired, or we experience pain, dizziness, or difficulty moving. None of these necessarily means that we have a disease, but we are likely to view them as problems that need treatment. Indeed, some people grow up learning to interpret many aspects of emotional distress as having a physical rather than an emotional basis.[10] And so we go to the physician or homeopath or chiropractor. . . .

How do we choose a therapist or therapy?

The choice of therapy brings us back to the subject of authority again. For most people, credentials are very important. But what are credentials? A Doctor of Medicine has credentials. A Doctor of Chiropractic has credentials, as does a Doctor of Naturopathy or a Doctor of Traditional Chinese Medicine. How is the public to choose among them? A Doctor is a Doctor is a Doctor to most people. When pharmacies promote herbal remedies alongside pharmaceuticals, when the nursing profession does not speak out against laying on of hands ("therapeutic touch"), and supposedly responsible media programs tout the benefits of unproven therapies, how is the public to choose among the various credentialed authorities? Not even looking for a basis in science is enough: Just as during wartime, when each nation proclaims that "God is on our side," so, too, do most promoters of therapy—whether conventional or alternative—claim science as their ally. Homeopathy, we are told, has passed scientific muster. Chiropractic is described as an art and a science and a philosophy. Say, which is that "scientific" medicine again?

Moreover, we happen to live in an age where there is, in many quarters, a growing distrust of established authorities. Today's distrust of authority is based in part on a devolution of social power that brings more and more decision making to the level of the individual, leaving less and less control in the hands of politicians, priests, physicians, and professors. On the whole, this is probably a positive development. However, when people are encouraged to make choices about health care, but are missing the tools they need to weigh one therapy against another, they are not necessarily better off, and may sometimes be much worse off, than when designated authorities made such decisions for them.

What if the therapist says there is nothing wrong?

What if the family physician informs you that the vomiting is due to stress and you should change careers, or tells you that your pain is just something that you will have to live with? Doctors are supposed to make us well. There is nothing in television advertising that says "Live with your headaches" or "There is not a pill for everything." If the doctor isn't making us well, then maybe we need another doctor. And if that doctor fails, then maybe we need another kind of therapy—at least one where they promise relief.

How do we know that a therapy works?

When we are given therapy for our problem, how do we know it works? I come back to where I started out, with the antibiotic. It works—we surmise—if we feel better. It works if our sore throat goes away or our backache improves or our warts disappear.

There are many reasons why we might feel improvement, however, even if the therapy has absolutely no effect. We may feel better after the treatment, even if it really had no effect, because:

- we were on our way to recovery anyway, or our symptoms fluctuate and we interpreted a temporary improvement as being due to the treatment;
- we never really had the disease—the symptoms were psychosomatic;
- we believed that the therapy would work, and therefore relaxed and slept better and ate better and helped our bodies along in that way.

Perhaps the therapy motivated other things that were helpful—e.g., given a natural medicine and told to avoid alcohol, we moderated our drinking; given a spinal manipulation, we came away feeling that the therapist really cares about us; given a herb, we mobilized the joint more, despite some initial pain;

• we want to believe that we are getting better, and so we reinterpret the symptoms and minimize their severity.

These and other factors (discussed by Barry Beyerstein in more detail in his paper in this volume [see chapter 6]) can lead us to perceive improvement in our symptoms as being caused by the treatment, thereby validating both therapy and therapist, and setting into play a new round of testimonials.

Incidentally, if "feeling better" is one criterion for judging a therapy as effective, what happens if we did not feel bad in the first place? Consider this: Research indicates that at least one-third of all patients do not comply with the medical regime suggested by their physicians.[11] Noncompliance is a particular problem when patients do not know they have a problem until they undergo a routine checkup. For example, even though hypertension can lead to stoke, heart failure, renal failure, and blindness, between 75 and 90 percent of patients diagnosed with this disorder fail to take their medication regularly or follow other recommendations.[12] Why such noncompliance? In part, it may be because the symptoms of hypertension are not usually obvious to the patient, who may wish to minimize the perceived threat by persuading him- or herself that there really is not a problem. This is a kind of "alternative nonmedicine"—if you feel all right, don't take anything!

However, there is more to it than that. The research literature shows that patients comply more when they regard their physician as caring, friendly, and interested in them.[13] Patients are also more likely to comply when physicians make definite follow-up appointments in order to monitor progress.[14] This again points to an advantage that some alternative therapists have over conventional physicians—increased specialization and technology and the economics of managed, third-party-payer health care tends to produce a rationing of the leisurely "bedside manner" that many patients crave almost as much as effective therapy itself. Alternative healers can cater to this need for reassurance, existential support, and sympathetic human interaction by being more friendly, chatty, taking more time, and scheduling a series of "maintenance" or "wellness" appointments. This in itself is not necessarily a bad thing, unless the alternative healer offers something dangerous, extracts unconscionable sums of money, or diverts the patient from proven therapies.

ALTERNATIVE MEDICINE
VERSUS SCIENTIFIC MEDICINE

So, when we ask "What makes people think that alternative remedies work?" we should first ask ourselves "What makes people think that conventional medicine works?" The answer to the two questions is pretty much the same. We think they work largely "because" we feel better after taking them, or authorities tell us that we are better. *Post hoc ergo propter hoc*—after the fact, therefore because of the fact. (Note that I am discussing the reasons for belief in a therapy, and not the efficacy of the therapy, per se). Proponents of alternative therapies are largely winning the public relations war with their hopeful, uplifting messages, whereas proponents of scientific biomedicine have so often assumed that the superiority of their product was self-evident (while underestimating the strength of the "antidoctor backlash" in society).

Alternative remedies have appeal to the extent that conventional remedies fail to provide relief. Indeed, the areas where alternative therapies seem to have most appeal is in the very areas where conventional therapies are not able to satisfy the expectations of the consumer—e.g., chronic headaches and backaches, low energy, nausea, arthritis, gastrointestinal complaints, allergies—things which are often caused by or exacerbated by stress or emotional disorders. The alternative therapist, through validating the client's complaints (and often his or her unconventional worldview), providing hope for overcoming the complaints, and giving much personal attention and support, can indirectly serve some of the emotional needs that often underlie many complaints that physicians dismiss. They also offer hope for conditions that physicians cannot cure.

Remember Chuanbeiye, the snake bile preparation I mentioned at the beginning? On the back of the box is written the following:

> This is an efficacious drug for sputum crudum, cough, asthma caused by cold, bronchitis and bronchitis chronic, etc. Because it is very sweet and convenient for taking therefore it is very welcomed by diseases at home and abroad. The effective rate that treats these diseases is 96.8 percent and the apparent effective rate is more than 76.8 percent.

That seems to suggest that some people get better but don't realize it! Whatever the author really meant to say, as patients with a disease, we have to leave it to medical scientists to establish the real effective rate. All our experience tells us about is the apparent effective rate—how often we seem to improve when we take the medicine, whether it actually helps or not. For the reasons I have discussed in this paper, it should not be surprising that alternative medicine is capable of producing "apparent effective rates" that are even higher in some circumstances than those produced by evidence-based medicine. Ultimately, therein lies their appeal.

NOTES

1. Beyerstein BL. Alternative medicine. Where's the evidence? *Can J Public Health.* 1997;88(3):149-150.

2. Gilovich T. *How We Know What Isn't So: The Fallibility of Human Reason in Everyday Life.* New York, NY: Free Press/Macmillan; 1991.

3. Schick T, Vaughn L. *How To Think About Weird Things: Critical Thinking for a New Age.* Mountain View, CA: Mayfield Publishing;1995.

4. Levy D. *Tools of Critical Thinking.* Boston, MA: Allyn and Bacon; 1997.

5. Alcock JE. *Parapsychology: Science or Magic?* Oxford, UK: Pergamon; 1981.

6. Alcock JE. The belief engine. *Skeptical Inquirer.* 1995;19(3):14–18.

7. Festinger L. *A Theory of Cognitive Dissonance.* Stanford, CA: Stanford University Press; 1957.

8. Alcock JE, Carment DW, Sadava SW. Attitude change. *A Textbook of Social Psychology.* 4th ed. Scarborough, Ontario: Prentice-Hall Canada; 1998.

9. Alcock JE. Chronic pain and the injured worker. *Canadian Psychology*. 1986;27:196-203.

10. Shorter E. *From Paralysis to Fatigue: A History of Psychosomatic Illness in the Modern Era*. New York, NY: Free Press; 1992.

11. Stone GC. Patient compliance and the role of the expert. *Journal of Social Issues*. 1979;35:34–59.

12. Leventhal H, Hirschman RS. Social psychology and prevention. In: Sanders GS, Suls J, eds. *Social Psychology of Health and Illness*. Hillsdale, NJ: Erlbaum; 1982: 387–401.

13. DiNicola DD, DiMatteo MR. Practitioners, patients, and compliance with medical regimes: a social psychological perspective. In: Baum A, Taylor SE, Singer JE, eds. *Handbook of Psychology and Health*. Vol 4. Hillsdale, NJ: Erlbaum; 1984: 5–64.

14. DiMatteo MR, Sherbourne CD, Hays RD, et al. Physicians' characteristics influencing patients' adherence to medical treatment: Results from the medical outcomes study. *Health Psychol*. 1993;12:93–102.

5

SOCIAL AND JUDGMENTAL BIASES THAT MAKE INERT TREATMENTS SEEM TO WORK

Barry L. Beyerstein

IF ONLY IGNORANT AND GULLIBLE PEOPLE ACCEPTED FAR-FETCHED IDEAS, little else would be needed to explain the abundance of folly in modern society. But, as James Alcock discusses . . . many people who are neither foolish nor ill-educated still cling fervently to beliefs that fly in the face of well-established research. Trust in the further reaches of complementary and alternative medicine (CAM) is a case in point. Paradoxically, surveys find that users of unscientific treatments tend to have slightly more, rather than less, formal education, compared to nonusers.[1] How are we to account for the fact that college graduates, and even some physicians, can accept therapeutic touch, iridology, ear candling, and homeopathy? Experts in the psychology of human error have long been aware that even highly trained experts are easily misled when they rely on personal experience and informal decision rules to infer the causes of complex events.[2,3,4,5] This is especially true if these conclusions concern beliefs to which they have an emotional, doctrinal, or monetary attachment. Indeed, it was the realization that shortcomings of perception, reasoning, and memory will often lead us to comforting, rather than true, conclusions that led the pioneers of modern science to substitute controlled, interpersonal observations and formal logic for the anecdotes and surmise that can so easily lead us astray. This lesson seems to have been largely lost on proponents of CAM. Some, such as Andrew Weil, reject it explicitly, advocating instead what he calls "stoned thinking," a melange of mystical intuition and emotional satisfaction, for deciding which therapies are valid.[6]

CAM remains, for the most part, "alternative" because its practitioners depend on subjective reckoning and user testimonials rather than scientific research to support what they do. They remain outside the scientific fold because most of their hypothesized mechanisms contradict well-established principles of biology, chemistry, or physics. If CAM proponents could produce acceptable evidence to back up their methods, they would no longer be alternative—they would be absorbed by mainstream medicine. It is my purpose in this article to draw attention to a number of social, psychological, and cognitive factors that can convince honest, intelligent, and well-educated people that scientifically discredited treatments have merit.

Those who sell therapies of any kind have an obligation to prove, first, that their products are safe and, second, that they are effective. The latter is often the more difficult task because there are many subtle ways that honest and intelligent people (both patients and therapists) can be led to think that a treatment has cured someone when it has not. This is true whether we are assessing new treatments in scientific medicine, old nostrums in folk medicine, fringe practices in CAM, or the frankly magical panaceas of faith healers.

To distinguish treatment-induced changes in some underlying pathology from various kinds of symptomatic relief that might follow any sort of intervention, there has evolved a set of objective procedures for testing the effectiveness of putative remedies. It is reliance on these procedures that distinguishes so-called evidence-based medicine from all the rest. Unless a ritual, technique, drug, or surgical procedure can be shown to have met these logical and evidential requirements, it is ethically questionable to offer it to the public, except on an admittedly experimental basis—especially if money is to change hands. Since most "alternative," "complementary," or "integrative" therapies lack this kind of support, one must ask why so many otherwise savvy consumers—many of whom would not purchase a toaster without turning to *Consumer Reports* for unbiased ratings from financially disinterested experts—trustingly shell out considerable sums for unproven, possibly dangerous health products.

We must also wonder why claims of alternative practitioners should remain so refractory to contrary data that are so readily available.

So, if an unorthodox therapy:

a. is implausible on a priori grounds (because its implied mechanisms or putative effects contradict well-established laws, principles, or empirical findings in physics, chemistry, or biology);
b. lacks a scientifically acceptable rationale of its own;
c. has insufficient supporting evidence derived from adequately controlled outcome research;
d. has failed in well-controlled clinical studies done by impartial evaluators and has been unable to rule out competing explanations for why it might seem to work in uncontrolled settings; and
e. should seem improbable, even to the lay person, on "common sense" grounds;

why would so many well-educated people continue to sell and purchase such a treatment?

Users of unscientific treatments fall broadly into one of two camps. Once a user of either stripe decides to try an unconventional treatment, and believes that his or her personal experience alone is adequate to decide if it has worked or not, the judgmental biases and errors discussed below have a strong tendency to make even the most worthless interventions seem valid. As Alcock points out in his article in this issue, users of the first type try unconventional therapies because they assume, erroneously, that someone else has put them to the test; i.e., they place misplaced trust in the usual authorities on whom they rely. They see an uncritical news item, receive a testimonial from a friend, or see a dubious product displayed alongside the proven ones in their local pharmacy. They may also overgeneralize from the occasional news report of an "alternative" treatment that has actually passed scientific scrutiny and been adopted by orthodox medicine.

The other sort of user chooses his or her alternative treatments out of a broader philosophical commitment. For users who choose CAM on ideological grounds, their fondness for these practices is rooted in a much larger network of social and metaphysical assumptions. Needless to say, their cosmological outlook differs substantially from the rationalist-empiricist worldview that underlies scientific biomedicine. Because these adversaries enter the fray with so few shared axioms and rules of evidence, it is not surprising that a consensus is rarely reached. Proponents of CAM disagree with their detractors, not only about the basic constituents of the universe and the nature of the forces that govern them, but also at the epistemological level—i.e., they cannot even agree about what are valid methods for settling such disputes.[7] Health being such a basic human concern, it is to be expected that differing opinions about the causes and remedies for disease would form a integral part of these two incommensurate worldviews—one objective, materialistic, and mechanistic, the other subjective, animistic, and morally driven. Because our views on health and disease are so enmeshed with our beliefs about the nature and meaning of life itself, not to mention the underpinnings of our moral precepts and our fundamental conceptions of reality, to attack someone's belief in unorthodox healing is to threaten this entire mutually supportive system of bedrock beliefs. Not surprisingly, such attacks will be resisted with strong emotion.

The ability to defend one's basic worldview is abetted by a number of cognitive biases that filter and distort contrary information. I shall return to these psychological processes that incline supporters to misconstrue their experiences to support their belief in CAM. But first let us examine the cultural milieu that has fostered a widespread desire to espouse such practices.

SOCIAL AND CULTURAL REASONS FOR THE POPULARITY OF UNPROVEN THERAPIES

As the twenty-first century [begins], several social trends have coalesced that enhance the popularity of CAM, in spite of (and to some degree, because of) its rejection by mainstream science. Today's resurgence of folk medicine can be traced, in part, to nostalgic holdovers from the neoromantic search for simplicity and spirituality that permeated the "counterculture" that attracted so many youthful converts during the 1960s and 1970s.[8] The aging flower children of the '60s and '70s now form the backbone of the "New Age" movement wherein unorthodox healing forms a central thrust.[9] Many of the "baby boomers" who spearheaded the earlier movement now find that CAM satisfies the mystical longings, desire for simpler times, and naive trust in the beneficence of "Nature" they absorbed during those tumultuous times. CAM also resonates with that era's mix of iconoclasm, reliance on feeling over reason, mistrust of science, and promotion of consumer advocacy. Let us examine how some of these features have promoted belief in nonscientific medicine among its clientele.

The Low Level of Scientific Literacy among the Public at Large

Surveys consistently report that, despite our overwhelming dependence on technology for our safety, nutrition, health, shelter, transportation, entertainment, and economic well-being, the average citizen of the industrialized world is shockingly ignorant when it comes to even the rudiments of science.[10,11] In a recent survey, only 52 percent of Canadians who were polled could say how long it takes the earth to orbit the sun! These days, it is quite possible to make it through college and even graduate school with virtually no exposure to science courses at all. Consequently, most people lack the basic knowledge and critical thinking skills to make an informed choice when they must decide whether a highly touted healthcare product is a sensible buy or not. When consumers haven't the foggiest idea how bacteria, viruses, prions, oncogenes, carcinogens, and environmental toxins wreak havoc on bodily tissues, shark cartilage, healing crystals, and pulverized tiger penis seem no more magical than the latest breakthrough from the biochemistry lab.

An Increase in Anti-Intellectualism and Antiscientific Attitudes Riding on the Coattails of New Age Mysticism

As a major plank in the New Age platform, CAM is permeated with the movement's magical and subjective view of the universe, epitomized in its catchphrase, "You create your own reality."[12] In advocating emotional over empirical and logical criteria for deciding what to believe, New Age medical gurus such as Andrew Weil and Deepak Chopra have fostered the attitude that "anything goes."[13] Even in elite academic institutions, there are strong proponents of the notion that objectivity is an illusion and how you feel about something determines its truth value.[14,15] To the extent that this has led many people to devalue the need for empirical verification in general, it has enlarged the potential following for those who sell magical and pseudoscientific health products.[16,17,18, 19,20]

Mind-body dualism permeates New Age thought, not least of all in its alternative medicine wing. Ironically, it is the New Age supporters of CAM who accuse their scientific critics of being dualists.[21,22] However, it is the CAM afficionados who are the real dualists, as evidenced by their constant appeal to undetectable spiritual interveners in matters of health. They need this obfuscation in order to support the oft-heard canard that scientific medicine undervalues the effects of mental processes on health.[23] The confusion this has spread in the public mind has paved the way for a resurgence of many variants of "the mind cure" so popular in past centuries; i.e., the belief that the real causes and cures for almost all disease lie in the mind, conceived by New Agers as coextensive with the immaterial soul.[24] It is easy to understand the appeal of such beliefs among those who have elevated wishful thinking to a virtue. Wouldn't it be nice if laughter and thinking optimistic thoughts would keep us healthy, prayer could rid us of diseases, or imagining little Samurais in the bloodstream attacking malignant cells would purge the body of cancer? Admittedly, there is evidence for psychological effects on one's health, but the size of these effects has been blown out of all proportion by CAM promoters such as Herbert Benson.[25] Several good critiques of the errors, experimental confounds, and artifacts that permeate the literature on spiritual beliefs and health have appeared recently.[26,27,28]

A related and troubling supposition common to New Age health propaganda is that one's moral standing can alter how forces in the natural world will affect us. In accepting this anthropocentric and animistic worldview, alternative healers are reverting to the prescientific notion that health and disease are tied to one's personal worthiness, rather than to naturalistic causes. This has fostered the return of an endless variety of long since discredited practices that purport to make patients "deserve wellness," rather than attacking the cellular bases of their diseases. Often, this merely leads to blaming the victim, for, implicitly, the patient must have done something despicable to "deserve" his or her affliction. And if the treatment fails, as it so often does, sufferers feel worse yet, for they must have been undeserving of a cure.

Vigorous Marketing of Extravagant Claims by the "Alternative" Medical Community

Strong profit motives have led alternative healers to promote themselves through aggressive marketing and intense legislative lobbying.[29] Routinely, promises are made that no ethical scientifically trained practitioner could or would make. In addition, new diseases of dubious scientific status are invented—and treated.[30,31] Unfortunately, facing this slick promotional barrage is a citizenry poorly equipped, in general, with the skills or information for evaluating this hyperbole.[32]

Inadequate Media Scrutiny and Attacking Critics

With some notable exceptions, the electronic and print media have tended to give CAM a free ride. The enthusiastic claims of the "alternatives," typically supported by nothing but anecdotes and testimonials, make uplifting stories that are all too rarely challenged by journalists who know that audience satisfaction cashes out in the rush for ratings.

Another disturbing trend that has had a chilling effect on some who would criticize unscientific treatments stems from the fact that many of these procedures have been imported from non-European cultures and championed by female practitioners. A rhetorical tactic that allows self-promoters to sidestep the substance of fair criticisms is to hurl accusations of racism and sexism at anyone who dares to express doubts; e.g., some practices, such as "therapeutic touch," that have been rejected by scientific medicine are being embraced by an increasing number of nursing schools. Because these are still predominantly female institutions looking to enhance the autonomy, scope, and earning power of their graduates by monopolizing new, sometimes dubious, spheres of practice, critics of practices salvaged from the trashbin of scientific medicine often find themselves accused of sexism. Similarly, when a colleague and I published a critique of several unsupported aspects of Traditional Chinese Medicine (TCM),[33] we were accused of cultural insensitivity and racism.[34] We were chided for presuming to criticize the effectiveness of TCM when we were not steeped in the philosophy of the culture that spawned it. To accept this absurd argument would be to agree that no one but a gourmet cook could tell when she's been served a bad meal. My rejoinder is, of course, that the truly racist and sexist attitude would be to hold empirically testable claims from other cultures or female proponents to a lower standard of proof than any others—this would amount to an assertion that their defenders are intellectually inferior. In the final analysis, appeals such as these to "other ways of knowing" amount to nothing more than tacit admission that these treatments cannot pass the standard procedures for vetting would-be therapies. Fortunately, since good science is practiced in the same way by all ethnic groups and both sexes, there are many strong opponents from within these communities who find ancient, unproven practices just as dubious as do white male critics.[35,36]

Increasing Social Malaise and Mistrust of Traditional Authority Figures—the Antidoctor Backlash

Growing disillusionment with the conventional wisdom and apprehensiveness about the future has fostered a certain crankiness in Western societies. This has intensified the willingness of many people to believe that our social, economic, and political shortcomings must be due to active connivance on the part of powerful, secretive cabals, rather than the cumulative mistakes of well-intentioned planners muddling through as best they can. Consequently, there is a growing desire to espouse grand conspiracy theories and to attack the institutions or interest groups that are suspected of plotting against the common good.[37] In this climate of suspicion, government is increasingly seen as a party to the plot and the scientific and medical professions have also begun to bear the brunt of what Richard Hofstadter identified decades ago as the "paranoid streak" in American politics.

These conspiratorial musings have coincided with two other, not entirely unjustified, undercurrents to promote an antidoctor backlash that CAM proponents have been quick to exploit. One is a sense of disappointment arising from the failure of certain overly optimistic predictions of medical breakthroughs to materialize. The other is the realization that medicine, as a self-regulating profession, has not always held the public good at the top of its political agenda.[38] This has added fuel to the social envy many people feel regarding the status, political clout, and earning power of the medical profession. As Ambrose Bierce once wrote, a physician is "one upon whom we set our hopes when ill and our dogs when well."

The inability of many people to separate in their minds certain self-serving actions of medical associations in the economic/political arena from the debate over whether scientific medicine's treatments are genuinely better than those of CAM has been a boon to the latter. In this fractious climate, the "alternatives" have also benefited by painting themselves as defenders of the democratic ideal of "choice." This would be commendable if consumers had the wherewithal to make an informed choice.

Dislike of the Delivery Methods of Scientific Biomedicine

There exists a widespread but exaggerated fear that modern medicine has become excessively technocratic, bureaucratic, and impersonal. The narrowing of medical specialties, the need to maximize the cost-efficient utilization of expensive facilities, the advent of third-party payment and managed care, and the staggering workloads of medical personnel have led some patients to long nostalgically for the simpler days of the kindly country doctor with ample time and a soothing bedside manner. They tend to forget, however, that this was often all a doctor of that era had to offer. Nonetheless, medical schools are coming to a renewed appreciation for the tangible benefits of interpersonal relationships in healthcare delivery and have begun, in their admission procedures, to look more closely at applicants' social skills in addition to their academic and technical excellence. The "alternatives" can rightly claim some credit for moving this up the agenda.

Safety and Side Effects

A quaint bit of romanticism that draws converts to New Age, "holistic" healthcare is the assertion that "natural" remedies are necessarily safer, gentler, and more efficacious than those of technological origin.[39] One hears frequently, for instance, the ludicrous claim that herbal concoctions have no side effects. If the ingredients in a natural product are potent enough to affect one's physiology in an advantageous way, they are certainly powerful enough to cause side effects as well. To say otherwise is to admit that one is administering an inert substance. In fact, some popular herbal concoctions are far from benign—a growing number of reports show allergic, toxic, even lethal, reactions among users of certain herbal remedies.[40,41,42,43,44,45] Numerous examples of mislabeling and serious contamination of popular herbal products have also been reported.[46,47] As usage rates rise, interactions with prescribed medications are also becoming more prevalent, since patients rarely know what is in the concoctions they are self-prescribing or receiving from herbalists. This danger is compounded by the fact that users are often reluctant to admit such indulgences to their physicians. Public awareness of the possible adverse effects of herbal concoctions has tended to be sparse because, unlike prescription drugs, there is no requirement that ill effects of supplements and herbal medications be reported to central registries. Unfortunately, under current U.S. law, the reverse onus exists, requiring the government to show that a supplement or herb is unsafe before manufacturers and vendors can be forced to remove it from the market.[48]

Among purveyors and users of herbs and supplements, even when adverse effects do occur, they are likely to be ignored or attributed to other causes. That is because there is a touching belief in these quarters that beneficent Nature would never pull such dirty tricks. In the same naive fashion, health food devotees staunchly maintain that "natural" Vitamin C from plants is more effective than the identical molecule manufactured in the chemistry lab, an idea equivalent to saying that bricks recycled from a cathedral will produce a better house than bricks salvaged from a brothel. Boosters of "natural" products should also be reminded that tobacco, bacteria, viruses, and prions are quite natural, too, and that some of the most deadly poisons known (e.g., belladonna, strychnine, cytisine, aflatoxin, and mycotoxins) are are found in wholly natural plants. On the other hand, over a third of all drugs routinely used in scientific biomedicine were derived from herbal sources, including many of the most widely used drugs in cancer chemotherapy.[49] The difference, of course, is that the active ingredients in these products, though originally from nature, are now known and have passed rigorous tests of safety and efficacy. This allows their purity and dosages to be accurately controlled, something than cannot be said of herbalists' products, whose active ingredients have been shown in lab assays to vary, in different samples, by a factor of as much as 10,000.[50]

Possible adverse consequences of other branches of alternative medicine have also been slow in being compiled, for similar sociopolitical reasons.[51] Fortunately, the Internet is beginning to provide some valuable sources of such cautionary information, though such warnings are in danger of being swamped by the torrent of hype and self-promotion on the Net. A number of websites containing scientifically reliable data about herbal remedies and supplements are listed in reference number 45, below. Similar listings regarding other aspects of CAM can be found at www.quackwatch.com and www.healthwatcher.net, the websites maintained, respectively, by Dr. Stephen Barrett and Dr. Terry Polevoy. Dr. George Lundberg, the new editor of the online medical journal, Medscape (www.medscape.com), has also announced that this electronic journal will be expanding its coverage of the possible harms of alternative treatments.

PSYCHOLOGICAL REASONS FOR THE POPULARITY OF ALTERNATIVE THERAPIES

Psychologists have long been aware that people generally strive to make their attitudes, beliefs, knowledge, and behaviors conform to a harmonious whole. When disquieting information intrudes and cannot easily be ignored, it is fascinating to observe the extent to which we can distort or sequester it to reduce the inevitable friction. It is to these mental gyrations that we now turn.

The Will to Believe

We all exhibit a willingness to endorse comforting beliefs and to accept, uncritically, information that reinforces our core attitudes and self-esteem.[52] Since it would be nice if many of the hopeful shibboleths of alternative medicine were true, it is not surprising that they are often seized upon with little demand for proof. Once adopted, such beliefs are remarkably resistant to contrary arguments. As Zusne and Jones[53] have emphasized, magical and pseudoscientific beliefs are typically parts of more fundamental systems of belief, ones that define the holder's basic concept of reality. Anything this central to one's cosmology and social outlook will be defended strongly, by filtering or misconstruing contrary input if need be.[54]

Logical Errors and Lack of a Control Group

One of the most prevalent pitfalls in everyday decision-making is to mistake correlation for causation. Logicians refer to this error as the *Post Hoc, Ergo Propter Hoc* fallacy ("After this, therefore because of this"). It is the basis of most superstitious beliefs, including many of the underpinnings of CAM. We all have a tendency to assume that things that occur together must be causally connected although, obviously, they needn't be. E.g., there is a high correlation between the consumption of diet soft drinks and obesity. Does this mean that artificial sweeteners cause people to become overweight?

When we count on personal experience to test the worth of medical treatments, we necessarily do so in situations where we lack complete information. The task of determining cause and effect is made even more difficult in the case of health care by the fact that many relevant factors are varying simultaneously—something casual observation cannot accurately track. This, plus the fact that the outcome of any single case could always have been a fluke, makes it virtually impossible to isolate actual causes when we base our decisions on personal experience in a single instance. Personal endorsements supply the bulk of the support for unorthodox health products, but they are an extremely weak currency because of what Gilovich[55] has called the "Compared to what?" problem. Without comparison to a similar group of sufferers, treated identically except that the allegedly curative element is withheld, any individual recipient can never know whether he or she would have recovered just as well without the vaunted treatment. Probably the single biggest failing of the CAM movement is its inability to see the need for the simple control group.

Judgmental Shortcomings

Those who cast doubt on fringe treatments are frequently dismissed with the rejoinder, "I don't care what your research studies say; I know it worked for me." It is well established, however, that this kind of intuitive judgement often leads to seriously flawed conclusions.[56,57] Unfortunately, the typical purveyor and purchaser of unproven therapies is insufficiently aware of the many perceptual and cognitive biases that can lead to faulty decisions when we depend on personal experience to decide what has caused a disease or whether a therapy "has worked" or not. Redelmeier and Tversky[58] showed how people are prone to perceive illusory correlations in random sequences of events. They then demonstrated how these intuitive feelings of association have led to the false but widespread belief that arthritis pain is influenced by the weather. Proponents of CAM, who take many folk beliefs like this at face value, seem oblivious to how easy it is to be misled by uncontrolled observations and misrecollections such as these.

The pioneers of the scientific revolution were aware of the large potential for error when informal reasoning joins forces with our penchant for jumping to congenial conclusions. By systematizing observations, studying large groups rather than a few isolated individuals, instituting control groups, and trying to eliminate confounding variables, these innovative thinkers hoped to reduce the impact of the frailties of reasoning that lead to false beliefs about how the world works. None of these safeguards exists when we base our decisions merely on a few satisfied customers' personal anecdotes—unfortunately, these stories are the "alternative" practitioner's stock in trade. Psychologists interested in judgmental biases have repeatedly demonstrated that human inference is especially vulnerable in complex situations, such as that of evaluating therapeutic outcomes, which contain a mix of interacting variables and a number of strong social pressures. Add a pecuniary interest in a particular outcome, and the scope for self-delusion is immense.

The job of distinguishing real from spurious causes in everyday situations requires not only controlled observations, but also systematized abstractions from large bodies of data. Dean and his colleagues[59] showed, using examples from another popular pseudoscience, handwriting analysis, that without large, sophisticated databases and statistical aids, human cognitive abilities are simply not up to the task of sifting valid relationships out of huge masses of interacting data. Similar difficulties would have confronted the elders of prescientific medicine, and for that reason, we cannot accept their, or their descendants', anecdotal reports as sufficient support for their methods.

Noticing interesting correlations in one's surroundings is a reasonable starting point for a systematic, controlled analysis that could actually reveal the underlying causal structure that might be exploited. Observing such a correlation, however, should never be the end point in a search for a relationship that could eventually be put to therapeutic use.

In defending their enterprise, proponents of CAM generally ignore these cautions and encourage instead another unfortunate human tendency, that of placing more faith in personal experience and intuition than on controlled, statistical studies. The "alternatives" encourage this in their followers by calling it independence of thought, which, of course, can sometimes be a good thing. They should know, however, that it can also lead the appraiser astray in many situations in which personal experience is not a good guide to the actual state of affairs.

Psychological Distortion of Reality

Distortion of perceived reality in the service of strong belief is a common occurrence (see Alcock[60] and his article in this issue of *SRAM* [chapter 4 in this volume]). Even when they derive no objective benefits, devotees who have a strong psychological investment in alternative medicine can convince themselves that they have been helped. According to cognitive dissonance theory,[61] when new information contradicts existing attitudes, feelings, or knowledge, mental distress is produced. We tend to alleviate this mental discord by reinterpreting, i.e., distorting, the offending input. To have received no relief after committing time, money, and "face" to an alternate course of treatment (and most likely to the cosmology of which it is a part) would be likely to create this kind of internal dissonance. Because it would be too disconcerting, psychologically, to admit to one's self or to others that it had all been a waste, there would be strong psychological pressure to find some redeeming value in the treatment.

Self-Serving Biases and Demand Characteristics

There are many self-serving biases that help maintain self-esteem and promote harmonious social functioning.[62] None of us wishes to admit to ourselves or others that we believe foolish things or that we are accepting people's trust and money under false pretenses. Because these core beliefs in our own virtue and intelligence tend to be vigorously defended—by warping perception and memory if need be—fringe practitioners, as well as their clients, are prone to misinterpret cues and remember things as they wish they had happened, rather than as they really occurred. In this way, therapists who don't keep good records and apply proper statistics (as is generally the case in CAM) can be selective in what they recall, thereby overestimating their apparent success rates while ignoring, downplaying, or explaining away their failures.

An illusory feeling that one's symptoms have improved could also be due to a number of so-called demand characteristics found in any therapeutic setting. In all societies there exists a "norm of reciprocity," an implicit rule that obliges people to respond in kind when someone does them a good turn. Therapists, for the most part, sincerely believe they are helping their patients and it is only natural that patients would want to please them in return. Without clients necessarily realizing it, such obligations (in the form of implicit social demands) are sufficient to inflate their perception of how much benefit they have received. Thus controls for this kind of compliance effect must also be built into properly conducted clinical trials.[63] Again, proponents of CAM downplay the need for such controls, possibly a form of self-delusion in itself.

WHY THERAPISTS AND THEIR CLIENTS ERRONEOUSLY CONCLUDE THAT INERT THERAPIES WORK

Although the terms "disease" and "illness" are often used interchangeably, for present purposes, it is worth distinguishing between the two. In what follows, I shall use "disease" to refer to a pathological state of the organism arising from infection, tissue degeneration, trauma, toxic exposure, carcinogenesis, and so on. By the term "illness" I will mean the feelings of malaise, pain, disorientation, dysfunctionality, or other subjective complaints that might accompany a disease state. Our subjective reaction to the raw sensations we call symptoms is, like all other perceptions, a complex cognitive construction. As such, it is molded by factors such as beliefs, suggestions, expectations, demand characteristics, self-serving biases, and self-deception. The experience of illness is also affected (often unconsciously) by a host of social, monetary, and psychological payoffs that accrue to those admitted to the "sick role" by society's gatekeepers (i.e., health professionals). For certain individuals, the privileges and benefits of the sick role are sufficient to perpetuate the experience of illness after a disease has healed, or even to create feelings of illness in the absence of disease.[64,65] Awareness of these dynamics can be quite minimal in the nondiseased patient who has learned, through subtle psychological mechanisms, to feel ill. A conscious intent to deceive is definitely not required.

Unless we can tease apart the many factors that contribute to the perception of being ill, or being improved, personal testimonials offer no basis on which to judge whether a putative therapy has, in fact, cured anyone's disease. That is why blinded placebo-controlled clinical trials, with objective physical measures if possible, are absolutely essential in evaluating therapies of any kind. Bearing this in mind, then, why might someone mistakenly believe that he had been helped by an inert treatment?

The Disease May Have Run Its Natural Course

Many diseases respond well to "the tincture of time." In other words, they are self-limiting. Providing the condition is not chronic or fatal, the body's own recuperative processes will restore the sufferer to health. Thus, before the curative powers of a putative therapy can be acknowledged, its proponents must show that the percentage of patients who improve following treatment exceeds the proportion expected to recover without any intervention at all (or that they recover reliably faster than if left untreated). Unless an unconventional therapist releases detailed records of successes and failures over a sufficiently large number of patients with the same complaint, she cannot claim to have exceeded the norms for unaided recovery. As noted above, without an adequate control group, any given practitioner will never know how his clients would have fared without his ministrations.

To be fair, the "alternatives" are correct that many effective treatments in conventional medicine are also aimed at symptomatic relief or strengthening the body's own recuperative mechanisms, rather than attacking the disease process itself. It's just that proponents of CAM offer little convincing evidence that their own unique efforts along these lines are particularly effective. Nonetheless, the "alternatives" can take some satisfaction in the fact that the debate they have provoked has spurred conventional biomedical researchers to seek more effective ways of stimulating natural recovery processes, such as enhancing certain immune reactions. Unfortunately, their disinterest in research means that the "alternatives" will contribute little to the understanding that will eventually lead to therapeutic improvements.

Many Diseases Are Cyclical

Arthritis, multiple sclerosis, allergies, and gastrointestinal complaints are examples of diseases that normally "have their ups and downs." Not surprisingly, sufferers tend to seek therapy during the downturn of any given cycle. In this way, a bogus treatment will have repeated opportunities to coincide with upturns that would have happened anyway. Again, in the absence of appropriate control groups, consumers and vendors alike are prone to misinterpret improvement due to normal cyclical variation as a valid therapeutic effect.

Spontaneous Remission

Any anecdotally reported cure could have been due to a rare but possible "spontaneous remission." Even with certain cancers that are nearly always lethal, tumors occasionally disappear without further treatment. One experienced oncologist reports that he has seen 12 such events in about 6,000 cases he has treated.[66] Alternative therapists can receive unearned acclaim for such remissions because many desperate patients turn to them out of a feeling that they have nothing left to lose. When the "alternatives" assert that they have snatched many hopeless individuals from death's door, they rarely reveal what percentage of their apparently terminal clientele such happy exceptions represent. What is needed is statistical evidence that their "cure rates" exceed the known spontaneous remission rate and the placebo response rate (see below) for the conditions they treat.

The exact mechanisms responsible for spontaneous remissions are not well understood at present, but much research is being devoted to revealing and possibly harnessing processes in the immune system or elsewhere that are responsible for these unexpected turnarounds. Some researchers think that spontaneous remissions are less the result of immune surveillance than the fact that certain biochemical reactions necessary for growth in malignant masses can, on occasion, reach a self-limiting stage before the accumulated tumor mass kills the patient. Whatever the mechanism, the documented existence of spontaneous remissions in a variety of diseases, in people who do not avail themselves of alternative treatments, means that an occasional dramatic, unexpected turnaround cannot be used to validate the power of prayer or a fringe therapy.

The Placebo Effect and the Need for Randomized, Double-Blind Assessments

A major reason bogus remedies are credited with subjective, and occasionally objective, improvements is the ubiquitous placebo effect.[67,68,69] The history of medicine is strewn with examples of what, in hindsight, seem like crackpot procedures that were once enthusiastically endorsed by physicians and patients alike.[70,71,72] Misconceptions of this sort arise from the false assumption that a change in symptoms following a treatment must have been a specific consequence of that procedure. Through a combination of suggestion, belief, expectancy, cognitive reinterpretation, and attentional diversion, patients given biologically useless treatments can often experience measurable relief nonetheless. Some placebo responses produce actual changes in physical symptoms; others are subjective changes that make patients feel better in the absence of measurable changes in their underlying pathology.

Through repeated contact with valid therapeutic procedures, we all develop, much like Pavlov's dogs, conditioned responses in various physiological systems. Later, these responses can be triggered by the setting, rituals, paraphernalia, and verbal cues that signal the act of "being treated." Among other things, placebos can cause release of the body's own morphine-like pain killers, the endorphins.[73] Because these learned responses can be palliative, even when a treatment itself is irrelevant to the source of the complaint, it is necessary that putative therapies be tested against a placebo control group—i.e., similar patients who receive a sham treatment that resembles the "real" one, except that the suspected active ingredient is withheld.

It is essential that the patients in such tests be randomly assigned to their respective treatment groups. Otherwise, sicker or more compliant people could end up in one group or another, or people with harmful or helpful lifestyles or certain habits, industrial exposures, and so on, could be disproportionately allocated. These group differences could produce effects that might be spuriously attributed to the experimental manipulation—something researchers call an "experimental confound." Good examples of the mischief such confounds can wreak are discussed in a recent critique of studies purporting to show that various religious practices enhance health.[74] Indeed, practicing members of certain faiths do seem to enjoy certain medical benefits. The question, however, is whether faith itself is responsible—i.e., a benevolent deity looks out for the pious—or simply that observant believers also tend to smoke and drink less, engage in fewer risky activities, live in less toxic environments, enjoy better social support networks, come from certain ethnic backgrounds, and so on. And, of course, given that stress can have adverse health consequences, belief in a supernatural protector could be health-promoting via its ability to alleviate anxiety, regardless of whether the belief is true or not. Once again we see the perils of assuming that correlation implies causation.

In addition, adequately controlled research requires that all recipients must be "blind" with respect to whether they are receiving the active versus the placebo treatment. Because the power of what psychologists call "expectancy and compliance effects" is so strong, the therapists must also be blind as to the group membership of individual patients.[75] Hence the term "double-blind"—the gold standard of outcome research. Such precautions are required because barely perceptible cues, unintentionally conveyed by treatment providers who are not blinded, can bias test results. Likewise, those who assess the treatment's effects must also be blind, for there is a large literature on "experimenter bias" showing that honest and well-trained professionals can unconsciously "read in" the outcomes they expect when they attempt to assess complex events.[76,77] If one's professional advancement or net worth depends on validation of a putative treatment, there is all the more need for blind assessments. Ideally, the end points being measured will be objective, and if the measurements can be mechanized and automated to reduce the effects of observer subjectivity, so much the better. It is odd that CAM supporters who would not think much of a wine tasting that failed to obscure the labels on the bottles still downplay the need for blinded assessments when it comes to their own stock-in-trade.

When the clinical trial is completed, the blinds can then be broken to allow statistical comparison of active, placebo, and untreated groups. Only if the improvements observed in the active treatment group exceed those in the other two groups by a statistically significant amount can the therapy claim legitimacy.

Defenders of CAM often complain that conventional medicine itself continues to use many treatments that have not been adequately vetted in placebo-controlled, double-blind trials. This may be so in some instances, but the percentage of such holdovers is grossly exaggerated by the "alternatives."[78] At any rate, this does nothing to enhance the credibility of CAM, for merely arguing that "they're as bad as we are" offers no positive evidence in favor of one's own pet belief. The crucial difference between scientific biomedicine and alternative medicine is that the former is institutionally committed to finding empirical support for its treatments and eventually weeds out those that fail to pass muster. And, unlike the "alternatives," biomedicine does not cling to procedures that contradict well-established principles in the basic sciences. Scientifically based therapies change because new research accumulates; alternative medicine is mired in the past and changes rarely, if ever. This is because the latter has no serious commitment to testing its rationales and procedures under controlled conditions. Alternative medicine clings to the belief that its procedures must be valid because they have stood the test of time. But the longevity of racism, sexism, and the belief in demonic possession belies the assertion that ability to survive implies validity.

Some Allegedly Cured Symptoms Were Probably Psychosomatic to Begin With

The pioneering neurologist Joseph Babinski (1857– 1932) coined the term "pithiatism" to refer to conditions he concluded were "caused by suggestion, cured by persuasion." A constant difficulty in trying to measure therapeutic effectiveness is that there are many such complaints that can both arise from psychosocial distress and be alleviated by support and reassurance. At first glance, these symptoms (at various times called "psychosomatic," "hysterical," or "neurasthenic") resemble those of recognized medical syndromes.[79,80] Although there are many "secondary gains" (i.e., psychological, social, and economic payoffs) that accrue to those who slip into "the sick role" in this way, we need not accuse them of conscious malingering to point out that their symptoms are nonetheless maintained by subtle psychosocial processes.[81]

Alternative healers cater to these members of the "worried well" who are mistakenly convinced that they have organic diseases or morbidly fearful that they may lose their good health. Their complaints are instances of somatization, the tendency to express psychological concerns in a language of symptoms like those of organic diseases.[82,83,84] The "alternatives" offer comfort to these individuals who need to believe their symptoms have medical rather than psychological causes. Often with the aid of pseudoscientific diagnostic devices, fringe practitioners reinforce the somatizer's conviction that the cold-hearted, narrow-minded medical establishment, who can find nothing physically amiss, is both incompetent and unfair in refusing to acknowledge a very real organic condition. A large proportion of those diagnosed with "chronic fatigue," "environmental sensitivity syndrome," irritable bowel syndrome, fibromyalgia, and posttraumatic stress disorders (not to mention many suing manufacturers because of the allegedly harmful effects of silicone breast implants[85]) look very much like classic somatizers.[86,87] Similar dynamics seem to underlie reports of a more recent variant of what Stewart[88] has called this family of "fashionable diseases," i.e., "Gulf War Syndrome."[89]

If a patient's symptoms were psychologically caused to begin with, he or she is likely to respond favorably to an acceptable blend of suggestion, reassurance, psychological support, and reaffirmation. Often this is what (probably unknowingly) these patients are really seeking through their illness behavior. In rejecting this interpretation, CAM practitioners ask why, if the malaise is really of psychological origin, wouldn't relief have been achieved already from any of the typically long list of abandoned conventional physicians? One answer is that the patient-doctor rapport necessary for such reassurance to be effective is likely to become strained as soon as the doctor says she cannot find any physical cause for the illness. If a physician even hints at a psychosomatic diagnosis, the relationship is likely to be poisoned irrevocably—for, sad to say, even in this supposedly enlightened age, psychological diagnoses still carry a social stigma for many. Thereafter, no amount of support and reassurance is likely to bridge the gap that has been opened. Curiously, though, when the alternative healer gives the sought-after physical diagnosis and then, in the next breath, reverts to the New Age line that all diseases are caused by mental/spiritual shortcomings, the same patient may well accept this about-face with enthusiasm. To the extent that alternative healers are often charismatic personalities who are willing to spend extensive amounts of time reassuring their clients and catering to their existential concerns, this heightens their ability to capitalize on patient suggestibility.[90] It also stands to reason that suggestions arising from someone who buys into the patient's metaphysical outlook might be more effective in countering psychosomatic complaints than those following from a philosophically skeptical point of view.

When, through the role-governed rituals of "delivering treatment," fringe therapists supply the reassurance, sense of belonging, and existential support that their clients are seeking, this is obviously worthwhile, but all this need not be foreign to scientific practitioners who have much more to offer besides. The downside is that catering to the desire for medical diagnoses for psychological complaints promotes pseudoscience and magical thinking while unduly inflating the success rates of medical quacks. Saddest of all, it perpetuates the prejudicial anachronism that there is something shameful or illegitimate about psychological problems.

Symptomatic Relief versus Cure

Short of an outright cure, alleviating pain and discomfort is what sick people value most. Many allegedly curative treatments offered by alternative practitioners, while unable to affect the disease process itself, do make the illness more bearable, but for psychological reasons. Pain is one example. Much research shows that pain is partly a sensation like seeing or hearing and partly an emotion.[91,92] Researchers have found repeatedly that anything that successfully reduces the emotional component of pain leaves the purely sensory portion surprisingly tolerable. Thus, suffering can often be reduced by psychological means, even if the underlying pathology is untouched. Anything that can allay anxiety, redirect attention, reduce arousal, foster a sense of control, or lead to cognitive reinterpretation of symptoms can alleviate the agony component of pain. Modern multidisciplinary pain clinics put these strategies to good use every day.[93] Whenever patients suffer less, this is all to the good, but we must be careful that purely symptomatic relief does not divert people from proven remedies for the underlying condition until it is too late for them to be effective.

Many Consumers of Alternative Therapies Hedge Their Bets

In an attempt to appeal to a wider clientele, many unorthodox healers have begun to refer to themselves as "complementary" or "integrative," rather than "alternative." Instead of ministering primarily to the ideologically committed or those who have been told there is nothing more that conventional medicine can do for them, the "alternatives" have begun to advertise that they can enhance conventional biomedical treatments. They accept that orthodox practitioners can alleviate specific symptoms but contend that alternative medicine treats the real causes of disease— dubious dietary imbalances or environmental sensitivities, disrupted energy fields, or even unresolved conflicts from previous incarnations.[94] If improvement follows the combined delivery of "complementary" and scientifically based treatments, the fringe practice often gets a disproportionate share of the credit.

Misdiagnosis by Self or by a Physician

In this era of media obsession with health, many people can be induced to think they suffer from diseases they do not have. When these healthy folk receive the oddly unwelcome news from orthodox physicians that they have no organic signs of disease, they often gravitate to alternative practitioners who can always find some kind of "energy imbalance," nutritional deficit, or dubious "sensitivity" to treat. If "recovery" should follow, another convert is born.

Scientifically trained physicians do not claim infallibility, and a mistaken diagnosis, followed by a trip to a shrine, alternative healer, or herb counter, can lead to a glowing testimonial for having cured a grave condition that never existed. Other times, the diagnosis may have been correct but the time course, which is inherently hard to predict, might have proved inaccurate. If a patient with a terminal condition undergoes alternative treatments and succumbs later than the conventional doctor predicted, the alternative procedure may receive credit for prolonging life when, in fact, the discrepancy was merely due to an unduly pessimistic prognosis. I.e., survival was longer than the expected norm, but within the range of normal statistical variation for the disease in question.

Derivative Benefits

Alternative healers often have forceful, charismatic personalities.[95,96,97] To the extent that patients are swept up by the messianic aspects of CAM, a psychological uplift may ensue that can have both short and longer term spinoffs. If an enthusiastic, upbeat healer manages to elevate the patient's mood and bolster his expectations, this enhanced optimism can lead to greater compliance with, and hence effectiveness of, any orthodox treatments he or she may also be receiving. This expectant attitude can also motivate people to improve their eating and sleeping habits and to exercise and socialize more. These changes, by themselves, could help speed natural recovery, or at the very least, make the recuperative interval easier to tolerate.

Psychological spinoffs of this kind can also reduce stress, which has been shown to have deleterious effects on the immune system.[98,99] Removing this added burden may speed healing, even if it is not a specific effect of the therapy. As with purely symptomatic relief, this is far from a bad thing, unless it diverts the patient from more effective treatments, or the charges are exorbitant.

CONCLUSION

Before anyone agrees to accept an unconventional treatment, he or she should ask whether it has been subjected to the sort of controlled clinical trials described above. As should be obvious by now, personal endorsements are essentially worthless in deciding the value of any therapy. Instead, supporters of unorthodox therapies should be able to supply empirical evidence, based on large groups of patients and published in refereed scientific journals. Only by this process of peer review can we be assured that the supporting research has been checked for the sources of error and bias described above. For example, reviewers look to see that the sample sizes were sufficiently large, the experimental design and statistical analyses were appropriate, and that obvious confounding variables were controlled for. The peer review process will determine that the participants were randomly assigned to treatment groups and that they were treated and assessed under double-blind conditions. It will also ensure that the condition of each patient was accurately assessed and documented before and after the intervention and, ideally, that the participants were followed up for a reasonable interval thereafter to gauge the duration of any beneficial changes. And, of course, because any single positive outcome could always have been a statistical fluke, replication by independent researchers with converging methodologies is the ultimate assurance. A single experimental result practically never settles an important scientific issue. It is the long-term track record that counts. And even with published papers that pass on the foregoing criteria, one should always look to see how large the reported treatment effects are. Beware of the "true but trivial effect." There are many statistically significant outcomes in research articles that are real but too small to be of any clinical use.

Any practitioner who cannot supply this kind of backing for his or her procedures is immediately suspect. One should be even more wary if, instead of peer-reviewed research, the "evidence" comes solely in the form of anecdotes, testimonials, or self-published pamphlets or books. To be credible, supporting research articles should come from impartial journals in the appropriate scientific fields, rather than from journals owned by associations promoting the questionable practice, or from the "vanity press," which accepts virtually all submissions and charges the authors for publication of their work.

If the practitioner is ignorant of, or openly hostile to, mainstream science and cannot supply a reasonable scientific rationale for his methods, the would-be buyer should proceed with caution. If the "doctor's" promotional patter is laced with allusions to spiritual forces or vital energies or to vague planes, vibrations, imbalances, and sensitivities, suspicions should also be aroused. Likewise, if the treatment provider claims secret ingredients or processes (especially if they are named after him- or herself), extols ancient wisdom and "other ways of knowing," or claims to "treat the whole person, not diseases," there is also good reason to question his or her legitimacy. If the therapist claims to be persecuted by the medical establishment, encourages political action on his or her behalf, and is prone to attack or even sue critics rather than answering their criticisms with valid research, alarm bells should begin to ring. Practitioners who sell their own supplements and other proprietary concoctions in their offices and stress the need for frequent return visits by healthy people, "in order to stay healthy," are also a cause for concern. The presence of any pseudoscientific or conspiracy-laden literature in the waiting room ought to set a clear thinker looking for the nearest exit. And above all, if the promised results go well beyond those offered by conventional therapists, the probability is that one is dealing with a quack. In short, if it sounds too good to be true, it probably is.

When people become sick, any promise of a cure is especially beguiling. As a result, common sense and the willingness to demand evidence are easily supplanted by false hope. In this vulnerable state, the need for critical appraisal of treatment options is all the more necessary, rather than less. Potential clients of alternative therapists would do well to heed the admonition of St. Paul: "Test all things; hold fast to what is good" (I Th. 5:12). Those who still think they can afford to take a chance on the hawkers of untested remedies should bear in mind Goethe's wise advice: "Nothing is more dangerous than active ignorance."

NOTES

1. Millar WJ. Use of alternative heath care practitioners by Canadians. *Can J Public Health*. 1997;88(3): 154–158.

2. Nisbett R, Ross L. *Human Inference: Strategies and Shortcomings of Social Judgment*. Engelwood Cliffs, NJ: Prentice-Hall; 1980.

3. Schick T, Vaughn L. *How to Think About Weird Things: Critical Thinking for a New Age*. Mountain View, CA: Mayfield Publishing; 1995.

4. Gilovich T. *How We Know What Isn't So: The Fallibility of Human Reason in Everyday Life*. New York, NY: Free Press/Macmillan; 1991.

5. Levy D. *Tools of Critical Thinking*. Needam Heights, MA: Allyn and Bacon; 1997.

6. Relman A. A trip to Stonesville. *New Republic*. 1998; Dec. 14: 28–37.

7. Beyerstein B, Downie S. Naturopathy. *Scientific Rev Alternative Med*. 1998;2(1):20–28.

8. Frankel C. The nature and sources of irrationalism. *Science*. 1973;180:927–931.

9. Basil R, ed. *Not Necessarily the New Age*. Amherst, NY: Prometheus Books; 1988.

10. Kiernan V. Survey plumbs the depths of international ignorance. *New Scientist*. April 29, 1995, p. 7.

11. Beyerstein, B. The sorry state of scientific literacy in the industrialized democracies. *Learning Quarterly*. 1998; 2(2):5–11.

12. Basil, *Not Necessarily the New Age*.

13. Relman, A trip to Stonesville.

14. Gross P, Levitt N. *Higher Superstition*. Baltimore, MD: Johns Hopkins University Press; 1994.

15. Sokal A, Bricmont J. *Intellectual Impostures*. London: Profile Books; 1998.

16. Stalker D, Glymour C, eds. *Examining Holistic Medicine*. Amherst, NY: Prometheus Books; 1985.

17. Barrett S. *Health Schemes, Scams, and Frauds*. Mt. Vernon, NY: Consumer Reports Books; 1990.

18. Barrett S, Jarvis W. *The Health Robbers: A Close Look at Quackery in America.* Amherst, NY: Prometheus Books; 1993.

19. Pantanowitz D. *Alternative Medicine: A Doctor's Perspective.* Cape Town, South Africa: Southern Book Publishers; 1994.

20. Ulett GA. *Alternative Medicine or Magical Healing.* St. Louis: Warren H. Green; 1996.

21. Beyerstein B. The brain and consciousness—implications for psi phenomena. *Skeptical Inquirer.*1987;12:163–173.

22. Beyerstein B. Pseudoscience and the brain: tuners and tonics for aspiring superhumans. In: Della Sala S, ed. *Mind Myths: Exploring Popular Misconceptions About the Mind and Brain.* Chichester, UK: J. Wiley and Sons; 1999: 59–82.

23. Beyerstein and Downie, Naturopathy.

24. Meyer D. *The Positive Thinkers: A Study of the American Quest for Health, Wealth, and Personal Power from Mary Baker Eddy to Norman Vincent Peale.* New York, NY: Doubleday-Anchor; 1965.

25. Benson H. *Timeless Healing: The Power and Biology of Belief.* New York, NY: Simon and Schuster; 1996.

26. Tessman I, Tessman J. Mind and body. *Science.* 1997;276:369–370.

27. Tessman I, Tessman J. Troubling matters. *Science.* 1997;278:561.

28. Sloan RP, Bagiella E, Powell T. Religion, spirituality and medicine. *Lancet.* 1999;353:664–667.

29. Beyerstein B, Sampson W. Traditional medicine and pseudoscience in China. Part 1. *Skeptical Inquirer.* 1996;20 (4):18–26. Sampson W, Beyerstein B. Traditional medicine and pseudoscience in China. Part 2. *Skeptical Inquirer.* 1996;20(5):27–34.

30. Beyerstein and Downie, Naturopathy.

31. Shorter E. *From Paralysis to Fatigue: A History of Psychosomatic Medicine in the Modern Era.* New York, NY: Free Press/Macmillan; 1992.

32. Beyerstein, The sorry state of scientific literacy in the industrialized democracies.

33. Beyerstein and Sampson, Traditional medicine and pseudoscience in China, parts 1 and 2.

34. Hui KK. Is there a role for Traditional Chinese Medicine? *JAMA.* 1997;277(9):714. (A reply by W. Sampson and B. Beyerstein follows.)

35. Knauer D. Therapeutic touch on the hot-seat. *Can Nurse.* 1997;10:10.

36. Thadani M. *Herbal Remedies: Weeding Fact from Fiction.* Winnipeg, Manitoba: Context Publications; 1999.

37. Robins R, Post J. *Political Paranoia: The Psychopathology of Hatred.* New Haven, CT: Yale University Press; 1997.

38. Starr P. *The Social Transformation of American Medicine.* New York, NY: Basic Books; 1982.

39. Beyerstein and Downie, Naturopathy.

40. Thadani, *Herbal Remedies: Weeding Fact from Fiction.*

41. Ernst E. Harmless herbs? A review of the recent literature. *Am J Med.* 1998;104:170–178.

42. Tyler VE. *The Honest Herbal.* 3d ed. New York, NY: Pharmaceutical Products Press; 1993.

43. Sutter MC. Therapeutic effectiveness and adverse effects of herbs and herbal extracts. *British Columbia Medical Journal.* 1995;37(11):766–770.

44. Carter, R. Holistic hazards. *New Scientist.* July 13, 1996, pp. 12–13.

45. Winslow L, Kroll D. Herbs as medicines. *Arch Int Med.* 1998;158:2192–2199.

46. Ko RJ. Adulterants in Asian patent medicines. *N Engl J Med.* 1998;339(12): 847.

47. Betz W. Herbal crisis in Europe. *Scientific Rev Alternative Med.* In press.

48. Winslow and Kroll. Herbs as medicines.

49. Ibid.

50. Ibid.

51. Beyerstein and Downie, Naturopathy.

52. Alcock J. The belief engine. *Skeptical Inquirer.* 1995; 19(3):14–18.

53. Zusne L, Jones W. *Anomalistic Psychology: A Study of Magical Thinking.* 2d ed. Hillsdale, NJ: Lawrence Erlbaum Associates; 1989.

54. Beyerstein B, Hadaway P. On avoiding folly. *Journal of Drug Issues.* 1991;20(4):689–700.

55. Gilovich T. Some systematic biases of everyday judgment. *Skeptical Inquirer.* 1997;21(2):31–35.

56. Gilovich T, *How We Know What Isn't So.*

57. Tversky A, Kahneman, D. Judgement under uncertainty: heuristics and biases. *Science.* 1974;185:1124–1131.

58. Redelmeier D, Tversky A. On the belief that arthritis pain is related to the weather. *Proc Natl Acad Sci (USA).* 1996;93:2895–2896.

59. Dean G, Kelly I, Saklofske D, Furnham A. Graphology and human judgement. In: Beyerstein B, Beyerstein D, eds. *The Write Stuff.* Amherst, NY: Prometheus Books; 1992: 342–396.

60. Alcock, The belief engine.

61. Festinger L. *A Theory of Cognitive Dissonance*. Stanford, CA: Stanford University Press; 1957.

62. Beyerstein and Hadaway, On avoiding folly.

63. Adair J. *The Human Subject*. Boston, MA: Little, Brown and Co.; 1973.

64. Shorter, *From Paralysis to Fatigue*.

65. Alcock J. Chronic pain and the injured worker. *Canadian Psychology*. 1986;27(2):196–203.

66. Roberts A, Kewman D, Hovell L. The power of nonspecific effects in healing: implications for psychosocial and biological treatments. *Clin Psychol Rev*. 1993;13:375–391.

67. Ulett, *Alternative Medicine or Magical Healing*.

68. Roberts, Kewman, and Hovell, The power of nonspecific effects in healing.

69. Ernst E, Abbot NC. I shall please: the mysterious power of placebos. In: Della Sala S, ed. *Mind Myths: Exploring Popular Assumptions About the Mind and Brain*. Chichester, UK: J. Wiley & Sons; 1999: 209–213.

70. Barrett and Jarvis, *The Health Robbers*.

71. Hamilton D. *The Monkey Gland Affair*. London, UK: Chatto and Windus; 1986.

72. Skrabanek P, McCormick. J. *Follies and Fallacies in Medicine*. Amherst, NY: Prometheus Books; 1990.

73. Ulett, *Alternative Medicine or Magical Healing*.

74. Sloan, Bagiella, and Powell, Religion, spirituality and medicine.

75. Adair, *The Human Subject*.

76. Rosenthal R. *Experimenter Effects in Behavioral Research*. New York, NY: Appleton-Century-Crofts; 1966.

77. Chapman L, Chapman J. Genesis of popular but erroneous diagnostic observations. *J Abnorm Psychol*. 1967;72: 193–204.

78. Ellis J, Mulligan I, Rowe J, Sackett D. Inpatient general medicine is evidence based. *Lancet*. 1995;346:407–410.

79. Shorter, *From Paralysis to Fatigue*.

80. Merskey H. *The Analysis of Hysteria: Understanding Conversion and Dissociation*. 2d ed. London, UK: Royal College of Psychiatrists; 1995.

81. Alcock, Chronic pain and the injured worker.

82. Shorter, *From Paralysis to Fatigue*.

83. Stewart D. Emotional disorders misdiagnosed as physical illness: envi-

ronmental hypersensitivity, candidiasis hypersensitivity, and chronic fatigue syndrome. *Int J Ment Health.* 1990;19(3):56–68.

84. McWhinney IR, Epstein RM, Freeman TR. Rethinking somatization. *Ann Int Med.* 1997;126:747–775.

85. Angell, M. *Science on Trial: The Clash of Medical Evidence and the Law in the Breast Implant Case.* New York, NY: Norton; 1997.

86. McWhinney, Epstein, and Freeman, Rethinking somatization.

87. Huber P. *Galileo's Revenge: Junk Science in the Courtroom.* New York, NY: Basic Books; 1991.

88. McWhinney, Epstein, and Freeman, Rethinking somatization.

89. Joseph SC. A comprehensive clinical evaluation of 20,000 Persian Gulf War veterans. *Military Medicine.* 1997;162(3):149–155.

90. O'Connor G. Confidence trick. *Med J Aust.* 1987; 147:456–459.

91. Melzack R. Pain: Past, present and future. *Can J Psychol.* 1993;47:615–629.

92. Brose WG, Spiegel D. Neuropsychiatric aspects of pain management. In: *The American Psychiatric Press Textbook of Neuropsychiatry.* Washington, DC: American Psychiatric Press Inc.; 1992: 245–275.

93. Smith W, Merskey H, Gross S, eds. *Pain: Meaning and Management.* New York, NY: SP Medical and Scientific Books; 1980.

94. Beyerstein and Downie, Naturopathy.

95. Joseph, A comprehensive clinical evaluation of 20,000 Persian Gulf War veterans.

96. Nolen WA. *Healing: A Doctor in Search of a Miracle.* New York, NY: Fawcett Crest; 1974.

97. Randi J. *The Faith Healers.* Amherst, NY: Prometheus Books; 1989.

98. Ader R, Cohen N. Psychoneuroimmunology: conditioning and stress. *Annu Rev Psychol.* 1993;44:53–85.

99. Mestel, R. Let mind talk unto body. *New Scientist.* July 23, 1994, pp. 26–31.

6

THE MISCHIEF-MAKING OF IDEOMOTOR ACTION

Ray Hyman

In 1992, I WAS HIRED BY THE STATE OF OREGON AS AN EXPERT WITNESS IN a trial of four chiropractors who had been accused of using a "Toftness-like device" in their practices. The "Toftness Radiation Detector" was an appliance designed by a chiropractor for diagnosing ailments. It consisted of a metal cylinder shaped somewhat like a thick soup can. At one end was a lens; at the other was a smooth plastic "rubbing plate." A handle was attached perpendicular to the middle of the cylinder. In practice, the operator would grasp the handle with one hand and place the lens against the patient's spine. While moving the device along the spine, the chiropractor would rub the fingers of his other hand back and forth on the plastic rubbing plate. As long as the lens was over a healthy part of the spine, the operator's fingers would continue to slide freely across the plate. At least that was the theory.

According to Toftness, when the lens came to a diseased part of the back, the operator's fingers would encounter increased friction and start to "stick" on the rubbing plate. The lens, he believed, was sensitive to a very subtle form of radiation that was emitted by portions of the spine that were in need of chiropractic manipulation. Toftness conducted seminars to train chiropractors in the proper use of his apparatus. He would then lease these devices to them for use in their own offices.

In January 1982, the United States District Court in Wisconsin issued "a permanent nationwide injunction against the manufacturing, promoting, selling, leasing, distributing, shipping, delivering, or using in any way any Toftness Radiation Detector or any article or device that is substantially the same as, *or employs the same basic principles as,* the Toftness Radiation Detector" (emphasis added). The United States Court of Appeals for the Seventh Circuit upheld this decision in 1984.

Although the chiropractors who were charged by the State of Oregon claimed to have abandoned the outlawed Toftness device, prosecutors maintained that they were guilty of using a Toftness-like device. Their particular derivative had been designed by one of the defendants, also as an aid for spinal diagnosis. It consisted of a block of wood with an embedded concave plastic surface. This time, however, the "rubbing plate" was placed on an adjacent horizontal surface, rather than being part of the instrument that was in direct contact with the spine. The chiropractor would use his left hand to palpate the patient's spine while he moved the fingers of his right hand back and forth across the plastic rubbing plate. In this slight variation on Toftness's theme, the defendants claimed that whenever their left hand contacted a problematic spot on a patient's spine, friction would increase, causing the fingers of their right hand to "stick" on the rubbing plate.

Despite these similarities, the Oregon chiropractors strongly denied that theirs was a Toftness-like device. Although the chiropractor who designed the Oregon rubbing plate had been trained by Toftness and had previously used the Toftness Radiation Detector himself, he claimed that he no longer believed that Toftness' instrument detected radiation of any sort. In fact, he now believed that the sticking of the fingers on the plate with both the Toftness and the Oregon instruments was not triggered by any physical signal at all. Instead, he argued that the sticking was a trained subliminal response of the chiropractor, evoked unconsciously by his or her accumulated experience in locating spinal problems. He claimed that, although the visual and tactile signs of pathology obtained from spinal palpation were often too weak to be consciously perceived by a chiropractor, years of acquired expertise in spinal diagnosis were stored in his or her unconscious. Supposedly, this expertise could be brought to the surface with the aid of the rubbing plate.

A VIDEO DEMONSTRATION

One of my tasks as a consultant and expert witness for the State of Oregon was to produce a video tape to illustrate the psychological principles that made the rubbing plate seem to work. For this purpose, I used two groups of student volunteers. I met with the first group and showed them the Oregon rubbing plate which the assistant district attorney had loaned to me. I also showed them a pendulum made from a ring suspended from a cord and a pair of dowsing (or "divining") rods consisting of two metal bars bent at right angles.[1] With one rod in each hand, I first demonstrated how dowsing works by holding the rods in front of me, aimed straight ahead and with their horizontal arms parallel to each other and to the floor. I then slowly walked about the room until the rods suddenly crossed one another. I walked away from that spot and showed how the rods uncrossed and became parallel again. I suggested that the place where the rods had crossed must be near a source of flowing water, perhaps a water pipe under the floor. I then requested that each of the students try the rods. To their amazement, the rods crossed when they walked over the spot I had indicated.

I then did a similar demonstration using the pendulum, before turning to the rubbing plate. I explained that the rubbing plate had been created by an Oregon doctor to amplify the sensitivity of our perceptions. To show how, I spread some playing cards face up on a table. I told the students that the red playing cards reflected mainly light from the long end of the visual spectrum. The black playing cards, on the other hand, reflected very little light, but what they did reflect contained an equal amount of radiation from all parts of the spectrum. Normally, I continued, the human senses cannot detect the difference between these two types of emission. However, by using the rubbing plate, we might be able to enhance our sensitivity to these differences, I suggested. I demonstrated this by passing my left hand back and forth, about a foot above the face-up playing cards. Meanwhile, my right-hand fingers were sliding back and forth across the surface of the rubbing plate. My fingers glided smoothly over the plastic surface whenever my hand was passing over a black card, but they would always begin to "stick" whenever my left hand encountered a red card.

I had each student try the experiment in turn. To their surprise, their fingers would also "stick" whenever their other hand was hovering over a red card. One of the students was from Africa. She became terrified when her fingers seemed to stick as her hand passed over a red card. She was convinced that this was the work of the Devil. I had to spend some time trying to reassure her that the sticking sensation was nothing but a normal, unconscious psychological reaction of her own, not demonic powers at work.

I did similar demonstrations for the second group of students. However, this time I let them see my dowsing rods crossing at a different arbitrarily chosen location in the room. Sure enough, for these students, too, the rods crossed just at the spot where mine had. Also, this time I told them that my fingers would stick only when my left hand was over a black card. As you might guess, for the second group, their fingers stuck only when their left hand was over a black card.

I made this video to illustrate a simple, but important, point. Under a variety of circumstances, our muscles will behave unconsciously in accordance with an implanted expectation.[2,3] What makes this simple fact so important is that we are not aware that we ourselves are the source of the resulting action. This lack of any sense of volition is common in many everyday actions as well as reports of those responding to hypnotic suggestions.[4] The latter report that their actions feel as though they are being propelled by powers external to themselves. My demonstrations with the divining rods had implanted the suggestion in each of the onlookers that the rods would cross at a certain location. When these students took the rods in their own hands and walked over the place where they believed the water pipe to be, they unconsciously made tiny muscle movements that caused the unstable rods the cross. They emphatically denied that they had done anything intentionally to make the rods move. Indeed, many insisted that they could feel the rods moving of their own accord, driven by some outside force.

The sticking response on the rubbing plate is even more compelling in this regard. When the students see one hand over the card that is expected to make their fingers stick on the rubbing pad, they unconsciously press somewhat harder on the surface and/or change the angle of their fingers slightly. This is sufficient to increase the friction between their fingers and the rubbing surface. The subjective experience for most students is eerie and they insist that they are doing nothing on purpose to make the sticking occur.

IDEOMOTOR ACTION

This "influence of suggestion in modifying and directing muscular movement, independently of volition" was given the label ideomotor action by the psychologist/physiologist William B. Carpenter in 1852.[5] Later, the concept was more widely publicized by the Harvard physician turned psychologist, William James.[6] Carpenter wanted to show that a variety of currently popular phenomena had conventional scientific explanations rather than the widely believed supernatural ones. The phenomena he tackled included dowsing ("water witching"), the magic pendulum, certain aspects of mesmerism, spiritualists' "table turning," and Reichenbach's "Odylic force." Carpenter did not question the reality of the phenomena, nor the honesty of the people who were involved. He only disputed the explanation, arguing that, "All the phenomena of the 'biologized' state, when attentively examined, will be found to consist in the occupation of the mind by the ideas which have been suggested to it, and in the influence which these ideas exert upon the actions of the body." Thus Carpenter invoked ideomotor action as a nonparanormal explanation for various phenomena that were being credited to new physical forces, spiritual intervention, or other supernatural causes. He published many books and articles during the latter half of the nineteenth century expounding his ideas about ideomotor action.[7,8]

William James[9] elaborated upon Carpenter's ideas, asserting that ideomotor activity was the basic process underlying all volitional behavior: "Wherever a movement unhesitatingly and immediately follows upon the idea of it, we have ideomotor action. We are then aware of nothing between the conception and the execution. All sorts of neuromuscular responses come between, of course, but we know absolutely nothing of them. We think the act, and it is done; and that is all that introspection tells us of the matter." James viewed ideomotor action not as a curiosity but as "simply the normal process stripped of disguise." James concluded that, "We may then lay it down for certain that every [mental] representation of a movement awakens in some degree the actual movement which is its object; and awakens it in a maximum degree whenever it is not kept from so doing by an antagonistic representation present simultaneously to the mind." Modern brain researchers have produced data and theory that help explain how quasi-independent modules in the brain can initiate motor movements without necessarily engaging the "executive module" that is responsible for our sense of self-awareness and volition [see chapter 5 in this volume].

Probably the first major scientist to become concerned about the mischief being created by ideomotor action, although he did not know the concept by this name, was the French chemist Michel Chevreul. Chevreul, who lived for one hundred three years, became interested in the experiments of some of his fellow chemists around the beginning of the nineteenth century. These colleagues were using what was known as "the exploring pendulum" to analyze chemical compounds.

The first recorded use of the exploring pendulum occurred around 371 C.E. A priest would bow over a plate, the edge of which was marked with the letters of the alphabet. This "diviner" or "oracle" would hold a ring, suspended from a thin thread, over the center of the plate. A question would be put to the priest. The movements of the ring would then be observed. When the ring was set in motion, it would swing toward one of the letters. This letter would be recorded; then the same process would be used to select another letter. This would continue until one or more words, which answered the question, would be generated. In this, we see the origins of the modern Ouija board, used to this day by occultists for divining purposes.[10]

In the early nineteenth century, certain chemists were advocating this method for analyzing the composition of substances. In 1808, a Professor Gerboin of Strasbourg wrote an entire book on use of the pendulum for chemical analysis.[11] As a budding scientist, Chevreul was intrigued, but he remained skeptical. He was surprised, however, to find that the pendulum worked as advertised when he tried it over a dish of mercury. He carried out more tests, however. To see if a physical force was responsible for the movement of the pendulum, he placed a glass plate between the iron ring and the mercury. To his surprise, the oscillations diminished and then stopped. When he removed the glass plate, the pendulum movements resumed. He next suspected that the pendulum moved because it was difficult to hold his arm steady. When he rested his arm on a support, the movements diminished but did not stop altogether.

Finally, Chevreul did what none of his predecessors had thought of doing. He conducted the equivalent of what we would call a double-blind trial. He blindfolded himself and then he had an assistant interpose or remove the glass plate between the pendulum and the mercury without his knowledge. Under these conditions, nothing happened. Chevreul concluded, "So long as I believed the movement possible, it took place; but after discovering the cause I could not reproduce it." His experiments with the pendulum show how easy it is "to mistake illusions for realities, whenever we are confronted by phenomena in which the human sense-organs are involved under conditions imperfectly analyzed." Chevreul used this principle of expectant attention to account for the phenomena of dowsing, movements of the exploring pendulum, and the then current fad among spiritualists, table-turning.

Chevreul was one of France's most prestigious scientists by the time he conducted these investigations. At about the same time, one of England's most famous scientists, Michael Faraday, published his investigation of table-turning in 1853.[12] By the 1850s table-turning (also called table-tilting or table-rapping) had become the rage among spiritualists, both in North America and in Europe. In a typical session, a small group of persons, usually called "sitters," would sit around a table with their hands resting upon its top. After an extended period of expectant waiting, a rap would be heard or the table would tilt upon one leg. Sometimes the table would sway and begin moving about the room, dragging the sitters along. Occasionally, sitters would claim that the table actually levitated off the floor. Table-turning was what first attracted many prominent scientists to the investigation of psychic phenomena. During the summer of 1853, several English scientists decided to investigate this phenomenon. Contemporary theories attributed table-turning to such things as electricity, magnetism, "attraction," the rotation of the earth, and Karl von Reichenbach's "Odylic force." Electricity, which the public at that time considered to be an occult and mystical force, was the most popular of these explanations.

A committee of four medical men held seances in June 1853 to investigate.[13] They discovered that the table did not move when the sitters' attention was diverted; nor did it move when they had not formed a common expectation about how the table should move. The table would not move if half the sitters expected it to move to the right and the other half expected it to move to the left. "But," the panel commented, "when expectation was allowed free play, and especially if the direction of the probable movement was indicated beforehand, the table began to rotate after a few minutes, although none of the sitters was conscious of exercising any effort at all. The conclusion was formed that the motion was due to muscular action, mostly exercised unconsciously."

The most publicized and carefully controlled study of table-turning was reported by Michael Faraday in 1853. Faraday obtained the cooperation of participants who he knew to be "very honorable" and who were also "successful table-movers." He found that the table would move in the expected direction, even when just one subject was seated at the table. Faraday first looked into the possibility that the movements were due to known forces such as electricity or magnetism. He showed that sandpaper, millboard, glue, glass, moist clay, tinfoil, cardboard, vulcanized rubber, and wood did not interfere with the table's movements. From these initial tests, he concluded that, "No form of experiment or mode of observation that I could devise gave me the slightest indication of any peculiar force. No attraction, or repulsion . . . nor anything which could be referred to other than mere mechanical pressure exerted inadvertently by the turner."

By then, Faraday suspected that his sitters were unconsciously pushing the table in the desired direction. However, his sitters firmly maintained that they were not the source of the table movements. And, as already mentioned, Faraday was satisfied that his sitters were "very honorable." So he devised an ingenious arrangement to pin down the cause of the movement. He placed four or five pieces of slippery cardboard, one on top of the other, upon the table. The sheets were attached to one another by little pellets of a soft cement. The bottommost sheet was attached to a piece of sandpaper that rested against the table top. This stack of cardboard sheets was approximately the size of the table top with the topmost layer being slightly larger than the table top. The edge of each layer in this cardboard sandwich slightly overlapped the one below. To mark their original positions, Faraday drew a pencil line across these exposed concentric borders of the cardboard sheets, on their under surface. The stack of cardboard sheets was secured to the table top by large rubber bands which insured that when the table moved, the sheets would move with it. However, the bands allowed sufficient play to permit the individual sheets of cardboard to move somewhat independently of one another.

The sitter then placed his hands upon the surface of the top cardboard layer and waited for the table to move in the direction previously agreed upon. Faraday reasoned that if the table moved to the left, and the source of the movement was the table and not the sitter, the table would move first and drag the successive layers of cardboard along with it, sequentially, from bottom to top, but with a slight lag. If this were the case, the displaced pencil marks would reveal a staggered line sloping outward from the left to the right. On the other hand, if the sitter was unwittingly moving the table, then his hands would push the top cardboard to the left and the remaining cardboards and the table would be dragged along successively, from top to bottom. This would result in displacement of the pencil marks in a staggered line sloping from right to left. Faraday observed that, "It was easy to see by displacement of the parts of the line that the hand had moved further from the table, and that the latter had lagged behind—that the hand, in fact, had pushed the upper card to the left and that the under cards and the table had followed and been dragged by it."

"IT'S NOT THE SAME THING!"

Faraday's report was sufficient to convince most scientists that table-turning and related phenomena did not stem from new physical forces or occult powers. Unfortunately, it inadvertently had the opposite effect upon a few prominent scientists such as Alfred Russel Wallace, the cofounder with Darwin of the theory of evolution by natural selection. Wallace had his first encounter with "the phenomena of Spiritualism" in the summer of 1865. He was seated with other sitters around a table. The table behaved in ways that he was sure could not be entirely explained by Faraday's findings and Carpenter's theory of ideomotor action. Faraday's research only dealt with one of the many possible causes of table movements. Indeed, in the original seances using tables, the movements were caused not by ideomotor action but by various cheating methods employed by fraudulent mediums and their accomplices. In addition, many converts' testimonials were obtained under conditions that tend to exaggerate normal human biases and result in sincere but mistaken reports of things that never actually happened.

Wallace experienced gyrations of the table that he was sure could not be handled by Faraday's findings. In his mind, this showed that skeptical scientists such as Faraday cannot be trusted to discover and fairly report upon truly revolutionary phenomena.[14,15] This tendency to dismiss a skeptical investigation because it cannot account for every instance of an alleged class of paranormal phenomena is what I call loopholism—the tendency to seek out each and every loophole in a skeptical account as a way to protect one's belief in a cherished supernatural or pseudoscientific claim. Wallace was familiar with Faraday's report. However, he seized upon the differences between the table's behavior in Faraday's experiment and what he had witnessed to assert that what Faraday had explained and what Wallace had experienced were not the same thing.

Perhaps the most striking, and saddest, example of loopholism is the story of the eminent American chemist, Robert Hare. Hare was professor emeritus of chemistry at the University of Pennsylvania when he became involved with table-turning in 1853, at age seventy-two. According to Isaac Asimov,[16] Hare was "one of the few strictly American products who in those days could be considered within hailing distance of the great European chemists." When Faraday's report was published, the *Philadelphia Inquirer* asked Hare for his comments. In his letter to the paper, on July 27, 1853, Hare firmly rejected the possibility that some exotic force could produce movement of wooden tables. He wrote, "I recommend to your attention, and that of others interested in this hallucination, Faraday's observations and experiments, recently published in some of our respectable newspapers. I entirely concur in the conclusions of that distinguished expounder of Nature's riddles."

A Mr. Amasa Holcombe and a Dr. Comstock replied to Hare's letter and invited him to attend a table-turning session. Comstock appealed to Hare's sense of fairness by asking him to observe and test the phenomena for himself rather than rely upon Faraday's report. Accepting the invitation, Hare attended a "circle" at a private house. He describes his experience as follows:

> Seated at a table with half a dozen persons, a hymn was sung with religious zeal and solemnity. Soon afterwards tappings were distinctly heard as if made beneath and against the table, which, from the perfect stillness of every one of the party, could not be attributed to any one among them. Apparently, the sounds were such as could only be made with some hard instrument, or with the ends of fingers aided by nails.
>
> I learned that simple queries were answered by means of these manifestations; one tap being considered as equivalent to a negative; two, to doubtful; and three, to an affirmative. With the greatest apparent sincerity, questions were put and answers taken and recorded, as if all concerned considered them as coming from a rational though invisible agent. Subsequently, two media sat down at a small table (drawer removed) which, upon careful examination, I found present to my inspection nothing but the surface of a bare board, on the under side as well as upon the upper. Yet the taps were heard as before, seemingly against the table. Even assuming the people by whom I was surrounded to be capable of deception, and the feat to be due to jugglery, it was still inexplicable. But manifestly I was in a company of worthy people, who were themselves under a deception if these sounds did not proceed from spiritual agency.
>
> On a subsequent occasion, at the same house, I heard similar tapping on a partition between two parlours. I opened the door between the parlours, and passed that adjoining the one in which I had been sitting. Nothing could be seen which could account for the sounds.

Hare goes on to describe other phenomena that he could not explain on the basis of normal agency. Although he dismisses the possibility of trickery, Hare does not seem to realize that he would find it just as difficult to detect the modus operandi behind a magician's tricks as he would to find a normal explanation for mediums' feats. In one instance, a skeptical lawyer friend indicated that what they had just witnessed must be due either to legerdemain on the part of the medium or to the agency of some invisible intelligent being. Hare's response is revealing:

But assigning the result to legerdemain was altogether opposed to my knowledge of his character. This gentleman, and the circle to which he belonged, spent about three hours, twice or thrice a week, in getting communications through the alphabet, by the process to which the lines above mentioned were due. This would not have taken place, had they not had implicit confidence, that the information thus obtained proceeded from spirits.

In other words, Hare rejects the possibility of trickery not because it was impossible but because people of "good character" would not have wasted their time on this if it originated in trickery! This same overconfidence in the belief that members of one's own high social class could not engage in treachery protected the often inept spy, Kim Philby, from being exposed for decades while he stole British and American secrets for the USSR. It also shielded the Soviet "mole," Aldrich Ames, who left numerous clues as he systematically plundered the files of the CIA for years.

Hare describes his subsequent research into spirit communication in his remarkable 1855 book which bore the equally remarkable title, *Experimental Investigation of the Spirit Manifestations, Demonstrating the Existence of Spirits and their Communion with Mortals. Doctrine of the Spirit World Respecting Heaven, Hell, Morality, and God. Also, the Influence of Scripture on the Morals of Christians.*[17] Before undertaking his research into spiritualism, Hare tells us he was a materialist and an atheist. He describes in detail the various experiments he conducted that, to him, proved the existence of the spirit world. He himself developed mediumistic powers. During these experiments Hare claimed he had communicated not only with the spirits of his departed relatives but also those of George Washington, John Quincy Adams, Henry Clay, Benjamin Franklin, Lord Byron, and Isaac Newton.

Hare created a device "which, if spirits were actually concerned in the phenomena, would enable them to manifest their physical and intellectual power independently of control by any medium." The Spiritscope, as he called it, consisted of a pasteboard disk slightly larger than a foot in diameter. Around its circumference he attached the letters of the alphabet in a haphazard order. An arrow that swivelled at the center of the disk was used to select letters one at a time by pointing toward them. For his initial test, he had a medium sit opposite him at a table. The disk was placed between Hare and the medium such that Hare could see the letters and the movements of the arrow but the medium could not. The medium sat with her hands on a surface above the table which, through a system of pulleys, cords, and weights, was attached to the arrow such that slight pressures of her hand would cause it to move in various directions and point to letters. Hare asked if any spirits were present. The arrow pointed to the letter Y (indicating "Yes."). Hare next asked the spirit to provide the initials of his name. The index pointed to R and then to H. Hare asked, "My honored father?" The index pointed to Y.

Hare carried out several more such experiments with similar results. Apparently he never fully understood the key aspect of Faraday's results—that honest, intelligent people can unconsciously engage in muscular activity that is consistent with their expectations. Although the medium sitting opposite him could not see the letters or the index on the disk, she was looking directly at Hare as he was observing the behavior of the index. We now know from many other investigations of ideomotor action—such as Oskar Pfungst's classic investigation of the allegedly intelligent horse, Clever Hans[18]—that people frequently give clues about what they are thinking or observing without realizing it.[19] These subtle clues can guide the behavior of other individuals—or even animals. Sometimes these individuals consciously detect these clues and use them to deceive,[20] but frequently the person being guided by the clues is just as unconscious of them as is the individual providing them.

Hare eventually found he could work alone, without the help of mediums, and still get meaningful communications from his Spiritscope. He had no inkling that he could be source of the messages being spelled out on his Spiritscope. Hare's example shows again that intelligence, professional accomplishment, and personal integrity offer no automatic protection against wishful thinking and self-delusion. Hare's Spiritscope served as the model for the later commercial development of the Ouija board—another striking example of the power of ideomotor action.

RADIONICS AND MEDICAL RADIESTHESIA

Perhaps in no other area has the seduction of ideomotor action created as much mischief as it has in medical settings. Over the past two centuries, many Europeans have used the term radiesthesia to refer to the alleged force that underlies dowsing and the exploring pendulum. The term is especially prevalent in connection with medical and healing applications. Medical radiesthesia is used to diagnose a variety of ailments—often from a distance. During this century, medical radiesthesia has often been merged with what is called "radionics." Radiesthesia remains very popular today among naturopaths.[21] Radionic devices are "black boxes" or similar contrivances that proponents claim have the ability to harness energy to diagnose and to heal illness. Today's practitioners of medical radiesthesia and radionics trace their beginnings to contraptions created by the San Francisco doctor Albert Abrams at the beginning of this century.[22]

Abrams had a conventional medical education, becoming professor of pathology at what eventually became the Stanford University School of Medicine. In 1910, Abrams claimed to discover that he could diagnose a variety of diseases by tapping his fingers on the patient's abdomen and listening for locations that yielded a dull sound. He then claimed to diagnose a patient from a distance by tapping on the belly of a proxy patient and using a drop of dried blood. Later, finding that an autograph was sufficient, he diagnosed by proxy numerous past celebrities, many of whom he diagnosed with syphilis. Next, Abrams built "electronic" boxes that would enable doctors to diagnose patients at a distance. He went further and devised other gadgets that he leased to others to treat patients at a distance. He required the others to sign an oath that they would never open them. But when finally examined, they revealed a functionless jumble of components. Abrams became extremely wealthy and earned an American Medical Association title, "the dean of the twentieth-century charlatans."

Some of his students had difficulty with the proxy percussion method, so Abrams devised a substitute—a glass rod drawn across the proxy's abdomen. When the glass rod encountered an area corresponding with the distant patient's disease, the friction would increase and the rod would "stick." Note that this "sticking" response resembles the modus operandi of the Toftness Radiation Detector and the Oregon rubbing plate. Indeed, Abrams was the grandfather of the use of the sticking response as the "output" feature of many subsequent radionic devices.

"Dr." Ruth Drown replaced the abdomen with a rubbing plate as the detection component in radionic devices. Mrs. Drown and her various contraptions were the objects of well-publicized quackery trials just before World War II. Like Abrams, Drown invented gadgets to both diagnose and treat patients from a distance. During the war, it became impossible to import Drown instruments into England. George de la Warr was recruited to construct a copy of Drown's apparatus for the British market, and developed grandiose and aggressively marketed descendants of the rubbing plate in England for 30 years. He added a variety of changes—all relying on a rubbing plate. He and his promoters claimed they had discovered a new form of radiation that would revolutionize science and society. In 1949, an inventor named Hieronymous obtained the first patent for a radionic machine. Not surprisingly, its alleged ability to detect unusual emanations depended upon a rubbing a plate and the sticking response.

FACILITATED COMMUNICATION, APPLIED KINESIOLOGY, AND TCM

Devices whose seeming utility depends ultimately on a rubbing plate or some related form of ideomotor action are still widely promoted on the fringes of medical, agricultural, forensic, geological, mining, and other applied fields. The preceding account provides the barest outline of the extent to which theories, systems, and machinery, dependent on some kind of ideomotor action, delude intelligent, sincere people—sellers and buyers alike. The following are three contemporary instances of ideomotor action in medicine: "facilitated communication," "applied kinesiology," and certain aspects of Traditional Chinese Medicine.

"In facilitated communication,"[23] the "facilitator" attempts to aid autistic children or those with other cognitive and language deficits to communicate. The child is placed in front of a keyboard, letters of which appear on a screen. The facilitator physically steadies the child's finger as it presses the keys. The child then types coherent sentences, apparently revealing high level communication skills.

Advocates of the method claimed that the children possessed high intelligence and considerable knowledge, but they could not express thoughts in speech or writing. Facilitators helped reveal the intellect within. Parents and many therapists were thrilled. Several university professors who specialized in treatment of mentally handicapped children claimed that the method was a revolution in the understanding of autism. Scientists who called for controlled experiments were rejected for showing lack of understanding and sympathy. Facilitators maintained that they were not influencing the children's letter selections.

Some patients, guided by facilitators, typed out messages claiming that their parents or other caregivers had sexually abused them. Reputations were ruined, alleged perpetrators were jailed, and families were torn apart. Eventually, controlled, blinded experiments isolated the information coming to the facilitator from that coming to the patient, proving the source of the messages was the facilitator, through ideomotor action.

Another example is "applied kinesiology." Legitimate kinesiology is the study of human motor performance using the standard tools of biochemistry, physiology, biomechanics, and psychology. "Applied kinesiology" purports to show that isolated muscle group weakness can be used to diagnose allergies, toxicities, and other disorders. Naturopaths and chiropractors are among its most ardent practitioners.[24] Such things as refined foods, foods grown with chemical fertilizers, artificial food colorants and preservatives, infinitesimal pesticide residues, refined sugar, or even flourescent lighting are said to sap vital energies and cause disease.

To measure susceptibility to such influences, practitioners place their palms face down on the hand or forearm of the patient who is told to exert an upward counter-force. The practitioner then puts a small amount of the allegedly offensive substance on the patient's tongue, skin, or nostrils, or turns on the fluorescent lights. The patient loses strength instantaneously, the kinesiologist's force easily overcomes the resistance, and the arm collapses. Of course, both participants in this folie à deux feel they maintain a constant effort throughout. As the reader is no doubt aware by now, such a demonstration proves nothing in the absence of a placebo control and a double-blind administration. Knowing an allegedly harmful substance has been applied, the practitioner unconsciously presses a little harder and the patient unconsciously resists a bit less.

Some years ago I participated in a test of applied kinesiology at Dr. Wallace Sampson's medical office in Mountain View, California. A team of chiropractors came to demonstrate the procedure. Several physician observers and the chiropractors had agreed that chiropractors would first be free to illustrate applied kinesiology in whatever manner they chose. Afterward, we would try some double-blind tests of their claims. The chiropractors presented as their major example a demonstration they believed showed that the human body could respond to the difference between glucose (a "bad" sugar) and fructose (a "good" sugar). The differential sensitivity was a truism among "alternative healers," though there was no scientific warrant for it. The chiropractors had volunteers lie on their backs and raise one arm vertically. They then would put a drop of glucose (in a solution of water) on the volunteer's tongue. The chiropractor then tried to push the volunteer's upraised arm down to a horizontal position while the volunteer tried to resist. In almost every case, the volunteer could not resist. The chiropractors stated the volunteer's body recognized glucose as a "bad" sugar. After the volunteer's mouth was rinsed out and a drop of fructose was placed on the tongue, the volunteer, in just about every test, resisted movement to the horizontal position. The body had recognized fructose as a "good" sugar.

After lunch a nurse brought us a large number of test tubes, each one coded with a secret number so that we could not tell from the tubes which contained fructose and which contained glucose. The nurse then left the room so that no one in the room during the subsequent testing would consciously know which tubes contained glucose and which fructose. The arm tests were repeated, but this time they were double-blind—neither the volunteer, the chiropractors, nor the onlookers was aware of whether the solution being applied to the volunteer's tongue was glucose or fructose. As in the morning session, sometimes the volunteers were able to resist and other times they were not. We recorded the code number of the solution on each trial. Then the nurse returned with the key to the code. When we determined which trials involved glucose and which involved fructose, there was no connection between ability to resist and whether the volunteer was given the "good" or the "bad" sugar.

When these results were announced, the head chiropractor turned to me and said, "You see, that is why we never do double-blind testing anymore. It never works!" At first I thought he was joking. It turned it out he was quite serious. Since he "knew" that applied kinesiology works, and the best scientific method shows that it does not work, then—in his mind—there must be something wrong with the scientific method. This is both a form of loopholism as well as an illustration of what I call the plea for special dispensation. Many pseudo- and fringe-scientists often react to the failure of science to confirm their prized beliefs, not by gracefully accepting the possibility that they were wrong, but by arguing that science is defective.

Another variation of this special dispensation was illustrated by the reaction of a dowser that Barry Beyerstein and I tested on an edition of the television program *Scientific American Frontiers*, hosted by Alan Alda. The dowser had agreed in advance to a double-blind test that he felt would prove his powers, but failed the test. Mr. Alda felt some compassion for this dowser, and discussed the failure with him. The dowser admitted he was disappointed but he felt that the outcome simply revealed that science had not yet matured to the point where it could cope with dowsing.

A final example of ideomotor mischief can be found in certain practices of Traditional Chinese Medicine (TCM.)[25,26] The essence of TCM is a scientifically undetectable vitalistic force called Qi (pronounced "chee"). Disease, according to TCM, results from an imbalance in the flow of the yin and yang forms of this universal "energy" in one's body. Acupuncture, Chinese herbs, massage, and so on, are supposed to restore the balance of Qi and thereby restore health. TCM practitioners claim to diagnose a wide variety of aliments using "pulse diagnosis" which bears little resemblance to the way scientifically trained physicians take a patient's pulse. The way in which the patient's hand is held by TCM practitioners while taking the pulse provides fertile ground for contamination by ideomotor activity (see the section on "muscle reading" in Marks and Kammann.) Not surprisingly, there is little to no objective evidence that these procedures have any diagnostic value. In a similar manner, TCM practitioners who employ the discipline called "Qi Gong" assert that they can direct their own Qi into others in order to achieve both diagnosis and healing. When a Qi Gong master's Qi is supposedly flowing, the "recipients" often feel suddenly energized or experience paralyzing weakness. In an unblinded demonstration shown on Bill Moyers' PBS series, *Healing and the Mind*, stalwart students were suddenly seen to lose the strength to push over their frail master. In properly blinded tests of Qi Gong masters, when "recipients" do not know when Qi is or is not being directed at them, such changes in how strong they perceive their muscles to be fail to appear.

SOME COMMON FEATURES OF IDEOMOTOR-BASED SYSTEMS

Although the effects of ideomotor action have been understood for at least one hundred fifty years, the phenomenon remains surprisingly unknown, even to scientists. To conclude, the following are some of the psychological features that characterize nearly all the systems and schemes that have bases in ideomotor action.

Ideomotor Action

To reiterate, all systems using the rubbing plate, the dowsing rod, the exploring pendulum, or related technique depend on an almost undetectable motor movement, amplified into a more noticeable event. The impetus arises from one's own subtle and unperceived expectations. Elaborate, grandiose theories are then devised to explain the observed effects.

Projection of the Operator's Actions to an External Force

This is one of key properties of ideomotor action. Although the operator's own actions cause the fingers to stick, the rod to move, or the pendulum to rotate in a given direction, the operator attributes the cause onto an external force. Subjectively, that is what it feels like. Lacking a sense of volition, one credits unknown forces, radiations, or other external emanations.

The Cause of the Action Is Attributed to Forces New to Science and Revolutionary in Nature

This is implied in the previous point. Not only is the cause attributed to an external source, but each time the phenomenon is encountered anew, those who have not read their history attribute it to a force previously unknown.

Delusions of Grandeur

Not only do the proponents insist that the cause is external, but they tend to see themselves as revolutionary saviors of mankind. They claim to have discovered new principles and forces, ones whose ramifications will transform contemporary science, not to mention society as we know it.

Delusions of Persecution

Those who suffer from delusions of grandeur frequently exhibit delusions of persecution. Self-styled revolutionaries assert that orthodox scientists dismiss discoverers of breakthroughs such as radionic devices and the like merely out of envy, pig-headedness, conformism, or unwillingness to give credit to brave outsiders who are not part of the scientific establishment.

To Be Forearmed Is To Be Disarmed

Proponents of quack devices and procedures will often argue that they are aware of ideomotor action and the role of expectancies. They often assert that their awareness makes them immune from its effects. Many dowsers now admit unconscious expectations can affect the action of the divining rod. They assert that their awareness prevents ideomotor action and allows expression of the "true dowsing response." Unfortunately, the awareness of ideomotor action does not make one immune from its expression.

Self-Sealing Belief Systems

Once the proponent becomes convinced that his favorite system "works," then the psychological forces discussed by James Alcock come into play. These self-serving biases serve to protect the belief system from falsification. Loopholism is one way proponents protect their beliefs in the face of contrary evidence. Saying "It is not the same thing" allows the believer to shield the system. Alcock supplies more examples of this ability to distort, forget, or ignore evidence. The true physician is aware of distortions of one's own judgement, as well as those of pseudoscientific competitors.

NOTES

1. Vogt EZ, Hyman R. *Water Witching U.S.A.* 2d ed. Chicago, IL: University of Chicago Press; 1979.

2. Ibid.

3. Spitz H. *Nonconscious Movements: From Mystical Messages to Facilitated Communication.* Manwah, NJ: Lawrence Erlbaum; 1997.

4. Bowers KS. Dissociated control, imagination, and the phenomenology of dissociation. In: Spiegel D, ed. *Dissociation: Culture, Mind and Body.* Washington, DC: American Psychiatric Press; 1994: 21–38.

5. Carpenter WB. On the influence of suggestion in modifying and directing muscular movement, independently of volition. *Proceedings of the Royal Institution of Great Britain.* 1852;1:147–153.

6. James W. *Principles of Psychology.* New York, NY: Holt; 1890.

7. Carpenter WB. *Mental Physiology.* London, UK: C. Kegan Paul; 1874.

8. Carpenter WB. *Mesmerism, Spiritualism, &c.* New York, NY: D. Appleton; 1874.

9. Carpenter, On the influence of suggestion in modifying and directing muscular movement, independently of volition.

10. Vogt and Hyman, *Water Witching U.S.A.*

11. Jastrow J. *Wish and Wisdom.* New York, NY: Appleton-Century-Crofts; 1935.

12. Faraday M. Experimental investigation of table turning. *Atheneum.* July 1853:801–803.

13. Podmore F. *Mediums of the 19th Century*. Vol. 2. New Hyde Park, NY: University Books; 1963.

14. Wallace AR. *On Miracles and Modern Spiritualism: Three Essays*. London, UK: James Burns; 1875.

15. Wallace AR. *My Life: A Record of Events and Opinions*. New York: NY: Dodd, Mead; 1906.

16. Asimov I. *Asimov's Biographical Encyclopedia of Science and Technology*. Rev. ed. New York, NY: Equinox; 1976.

17. Hare R. *Experimental Investigation of the Spirit Manifestations, Demostrating the Existence of Spirits and Their Communication With Mortals: Doctrine of the Spirit World Respecting Heaven, Hell, Morality, and God*. New York, NY: Partridge and Brittan; 1855.

18. Pfungst O. *Clever Hans*. New York, NY: Hold, Rinehart and Winston; 1965. [This is a reprint of the original 1911 edition. It contains a useful introduction by Robert Rosenthal.]

19. Hyman R. Cold reading: how to convince strangers that you know all about them. *Zetetic*. 1977;1(2):18–37.

20. Marks D, Kammann R. *The Psychology of the Psychic*. Amherst, NY: Prometheus Books; 1980.

21. Beyerstein B, Downie S. Naturopathy. *Scientific Rev Alternative Med*. 1998;2(1):20–28.

22. Armstrong D, Armstrong SM. The body electric: future shocks. In: *The Great American Medicine Show*. New York, NY: Prentice Hall; 1991.

23. Dillon K. Facilitated communication, autism, and Ouija. *Skeptical Inquirer*. 1993;17(3):281–287.

24. Beyerstein B, Sampson W. Traditional medicine and pseudoscience in China: a report of the second CSICOP delegation. Part 1. *Skeptical Inquirer*. 1996;20(4):18–26.

25. Ibid.

26. Sampson W, Beyerstein B. Traditional medicine and pseudoscience in China: a report of the second CSICOP delegation. Part 2. *Skeptical Inquirer*. 1996;20(5):27–34.

THERAPIES
AND
THEORIES

7

ANDREW WEIL
Public Perception and Reality

Arnold S. Relman

I

ANDREW WELL, M.D., IS VARIOUSLY DESCRIBED ON THE COVERS OF HIS best-selling books as "the guru of alternative medicine," "one of the most skilled, articulate, and important leaders in the field of health and healing," "a pioneer in the medicine of the future," and "an extraordinary phenomenon." On his website, which records over two and a half million hits a month, he is called "America's most trusted medical expert." A recent cover of *Time*, which featured the familiar picture of his bald head and bewhiskered cherubic countenance, announced that "medicine man Dr. Andrew Weil has made New Age remedies popular." In the accompanying story, *Time* tells us that "millions of Americans swear by" his medical advice.

Not all of this is hype. Weil is arguably the best known and most influential of the many physicianwriters now in the vanguard of the alternative medicine movement. He is also one of the most prolific. Since 1972 he has written eight books. The first three were mostly about the effects of natural drugs on consciousness, but the remaining five, all pub-

Originally published in the *New Republic*, 14 December 1998. Copyright © *New Republic*. Reprinted with permission.

lished in the past fifteen years, are about health and healing. Read together with one remarkable chapter in his first book, these more recent works provide a comprehensive description of alternative medicine, as seen through the eyes of its most serious and systematic advocate.

If Deepak Chopra is the mystical poet-laureate of the movement, then Weil is its heavy-duty theoretician and apologist. He directs a large and astonishingly successful medical marketing enterprise that might be called Dr. Andrew Weil, Inc. No longer the angry young rebel, he has become the urbane and supremely self-assured CEO of alternative medicine, who is seeking to reshape the medical establishment that he once scorned. The popularity of his teachings, and the spreading wave of interest in alternative remedies that he and others have inspired, are forcing mainstream medicine to deal with a counterculture that it would have preferred to ignore,

"Alternative medicine" is the term generally used to designate a varied collection of methods for the prevention, the diagnosis, or the treatment of disease that are not generally accepted by regular (or "allopathic") physicians and have not been part of the standard medical school curriculum in the United States. Some of these methods are very old. Acupuncture and other kinds of traditional Chinese medicine, as well as the Ayurvedic medicine of ancient Hinduism, were practiced before the Christian era, and they still flourish. Native American shamans and medicine men used herbal and ritual healing before the European conquest of America, and such practices still exist. In the nineteenth and early twentieth centuries, many healing cults were contending with allopathic physicians for popular support. These included homeopathy, naturopathy, and herbal medicine, psychic and faith healing, magnetic therapy and chiropracty and osteopathy. More recent twentieth-century additions to the alternative medicine family include therapeutic touch, guided imagery, biofeedback, and various forms of diet therapy. In the past few years, two new terms have come into use: "complementary medicine" and "integrative medicine." They identify a recent development in the alternative medicine movement championed by Weil and others: the idea that alternative medicine should be used in conjunction with, rather than instead of, mainstream allopathic methods.

Until now, alternative medicine has generally been rejected by medical scientists and educators, and by most practicing physicians. The reasons are many, but the most important reason is the difference in mentality between the alternative practitioners and the medical establishment. The leaders of the establishment believe in the scientific method, and in the rule of evidence, and in the laws of physics, chemistry, and biology upon which the modern view of nature is based. Alternative practitioners either do not seem to care about science or explicitly reject its premises. Their methods are often based on notions totally at odds with science, common sense, and modern conceptions of the structure and the function of the human body. In advancing their claims, they do not appear to recognize the need for objective evidence, asserting that the intuitions and the personal beliefs of patients and heaters are all that is needed to validate their methods. One might have expected such thinking to alienate most people in a technologically advanced society such as ours; but the alternative medicine movement and the popularity of gurus such as Weil are growing rapidly.

Weil's writings are ambiguous about the conflict between science and alternative medicine, as they are about many other issues in alternative medicine. Yes, he thinks that all healing methods ought to be tested; and yes, modern science can make useful contributions to our understanding of health and disease. Yet the scientific method is not for Weil, the only way, or even the best way, to learn about nature and the human body. Many important truths are intuitively evident and do not need scientific support, even when they seem to contradict logic. Conventional science-based medicine has its uses, but they are limited. Like so many of the other gurus of alternative medicine, Weil is not bothered by logical contradictions in his argument, or encumbered by a need to search for objective evidence.

This habit of thought was evident early in Weil's career. He was educated at Harvard College and Harvard Medical School in the 1960s, but he revolted against those academic bastions. Like many other students of his generation, he experimented with mind-altering drugs. He was a botany major and, not surprisingly for those days, he became interested in the psychedelic properties of certain plants. Later, in medical school, he participated in studies of the clinical and psychological effects of marijuana, which led to a few publications in scientific journals. He also developed a strong antipathy toward many of the basic concepts of conventional medicine, and the traditional pedagogical methods then employed to teach them.

We learn a little about Weil's postgraduate years from the brief autobiographical comments in the preface to The Natural Mind, his first book. After a one-year internship at Mount Zion Hospital in San Francisco in 1968–69, he began what was supposed to have been a two-year tour of duty at the National Institute of Mental Health. He resigned after a year. He says it was because of official opposition to his work with marijuana. He then left the world of allopathic medicine entirely, to go off to an Indian reservation in South Dakota to study with a Sioux medicine man and learn about herbal medicine and ritual healing. "On the reservation," he says, "I participated in sweat lodge ceremonies, grew a beard, and 'dropped out.' " At home afterward, "I started to practice yoga, experiment with vegetarianism, and learn to meditate." In 1971 he began to write The Natural Mind, which became a best-seller and launched his career as a writer.

The Natural Mind (1972) is mainly a criticism of American drug policy and an exposition of Weil's views on the interaction of psychedelic drugs with the mind. It also expounds his general philosophy of mind-body relations upon which much of his later writings on health and healing is based. The seventh chapter, entitled "A Trip to Stonesville," should be required reading for all who would understand the origins of Weil's belief in the healing power of the mind. It is a startling document—a sharply drawn manifesto of New Age biology, a direct challenge to the scientific basis of conventional medicine, and a revealing window on Weil's style of thought. And, since a theory of mind-body relations is central to most current formulations of alternative medicine, this chapter must be considered one of effective drug for high blood pressure." Now, even In 1972, when The Natural Mind was first published, this statement was dubious, to say the least; and it was certainly false in 1985 when the book was republished and supposedly updated. Weil tells us that patients can be taught to lower their blood pressure by a form of training called "feedback control." The fact is that "feedback control" (or "the relaxation response," as it is called by Dr. Herbert Benson, its chief advocate and another well-known guru of alternative medicine) produces at most only small and usually transient reductions in blood pressure. Feedback control has never been shown to be as effective in the long-term control of moderate to severe hypertension as any of a variety of pharmacological agents prescribed for this purpose. There are always risks of side effects with any active pharmaceutical, and antihypertensive agents are no exception. When properly used, however, they have proven beyond reasonable doubt to be a major advance in medical therapeutics. In fact, they are one big reason for the significant decline over the past three decades in the incidence of stroke, heart failure, and kidney failure, all of which can result from uncontrolled, severe hypertension. Weil would have been correct if he had simply observed that antihypertensive drugs are often used excessively, particularly when blood pressure is only mildly elevated. He would also have been correct had he suggested that a reduction in stress and a change in diet and lifestyle will often help in the management of such cases. But in *The Natural Mind* he suggests that self-treatment is the treatment of choice in many if not most cases. In his more recent books about self-healing approaches to health care, he is more prudent: he advises patients to check their own blood pressure and to seek guidance from an allopathic physician if simple remedies are not working. Unfortunately, the antiallopathic thrust in his teaching is more apt to be heeded than his cautions and his qualifications. Seriously hypertensive patients who delay seeking proper medical treatment may, as a result, suffer great harm. The neglect of available and often effective standard medical treatment for many kinds of illness would seem to be an inevitable consequence of the dogma promulgated in the seventh chapter of *The Natural Mind*.

Here are other examples of Weil's casual dismissal of common sense and medical fact in this chapter, and of his penchant for sweeping generalizations that cannot stand analysis. "My intuitions about disease are: first, that its physical manifestations are mostly caused by nonmaterial factors, in particular by unnatural restraints placed on the unconscious mind; and second, that the limits to what human consciousness can cause in the physical body are far beyond where most of us imagine them." Or, again: "Since leaving the world of allopathic practice, I have witnessed a number of impressive nonallopathic cures of . . . dramatic illnesses, including cancer and life-threatening infections." And later: "To the straight mind nonallopathic healing sounds very mystical. Faith healing is held in contempt by most rational people, despite the abundant evidence of cures."

Weil's later books make many claims for such "cures," as we shall see, but despite his reference to "abundant evidence," he almost never gives us anything more than the claim itself—unsupported by objective and documented observations. To Weil, subjective belief, if persuasive enough to the patient should be adequate to support the claim of reality. And by "reality" he does not refer simply to the patient's state of mind, but to the physical dimensions of the disease itself. The allegedly miraculous "cures" are not simply dramatic improvements in symptoms, but the disappearance of all physical evidence of disease. And why shouldn't this be reasonable if one believes, like Weil, that consciousness is the primary reality and that the physical aspects of disease, indeed the entire material world itself, are simply another aspect of mind?

The extent to which Weil reveres consciousness regardless of its thought content is revealed in the final sections of his "Stonesville" chapter. Here he favors us with his views on psychosis, on the Jungian theory of shared universal consciousness, and on the reality of mental telepathy, extrasensory perception, and hallucinatory experiences. On psychosis: "Psychotics are persons whose nonordinary experience is exceptionally strong . . . every psychotic is a potential sage or healer." With regard to the National Institute of Mental Health's research efforts to find the physical basis of psychosis: "If it sticks to its present course, NIMH will be the last institution in America to recognize the positive potential of psychosis—a potential so overwhelming that I am almost tempted to call psychotics the evolutionary vanguard of our species. They possess the secret of changing reality by changing the mind; if they can learn to use that talent for positive ends, there are no limits to what they can accomplish." With respect to C. G. Jung's ideas, Well says: "It appears that at some level of the unconscious we pass beyond personal awareness into a universal awareness unlimited by time and space. Most of us may think we never experience such a thing, but it may be that we simply never pay attention to it. I am convinced it happens." He then cites examples of such experiences caused by the ingestion of hallucinogenic herbs in Indian sacramental rituals. About shared consciousness and mental telepathy, he has this to say: "Not only do I think each of us can share consciousness, I think all of us are already doing it all the time. . . . Extrasensory perceptions are not unusual talents possessed by specially gifted individuals. They are normal unconscious events, and scientists who attempt to document them by laboratory experiments will never get to experience them directly."

One might think that this kind of talk, written more than twenty-five years ago by a youthful and angry rebel against medical scientific orthodoxy, would be an embarrassment to the fifty-six-year-old leader of a movement that aspires to integrate alternative concepts into the curriculum and the practice of conventional medicine. Not so. In a brief preface to the edition of *The Natural Mind* that appeared this year, Weil explicitly reaffirms his early views: "The philosophy of my first book is the same philosophy that underlies my writing about health." To be even more specific, he adds: "The seed of my thinking about conventional and alternative medicine can be found in chapter 7 of this book."

So we must take him at his word: he really does believe in miracles and in faith healing, in the ability of mind to cause and to cure disease, and in the existence of a consciousness that is in some real sense independent of the brain. In fact, these ideas reverberate in all of his later writing. The seventh chapter of *The Natural Mind* is simply the first and most forceful statement of a philosophy that has softened and blurred a bit, as Weil's career has progressed, but is fundamentally unchanged. And this philosophy poses serious intellectual problems for Weil's current attempt to integrate alternative and conventional medical practices.

II

The Natural Mind was followed by two more popular books about consciousness and mind-altering drugs—*The Marriage of the Sun and Moon: A Quest for Unity in Consciousness* (1980); and, with Winifred Rosen, *From Chocolate to Morphine: Everything You Need to Know About Mind-Altering Drugs* (1983). Neither book dealt directly with alternative medicine. His next book on medicine was *Health and Healing* (1983, republished in 1998). By then Weil had established himself in Tucson as a general medical practitioner and was on the part-time clinical faculty of the College of Medicine of the University of Arizona, where he gave an elective course of lectures about alternative medicine.

Health and Healing was the first of a series of five books he was to write in the years from 1983 to 1998 and, like most of them, it was a national best-seller. It established Weil as a leading figure in the alternative medicine movement. More than any of his writings before or after, it provided a broad and fairly systematic exposition of his opinions on the nature of health and healing, on allopathic medicine, and on the varieties of alternative or unconventional medicine. In the preface to the 1998 edition of *Health and Healing*, Weil remarks that "it remains the philosophical and theoretical basis of all my subsequent work in medicine."

Consider Weil's strange discussion in this book of sickness and health. "Sickness is the manifestation of evil in the body," he proclaims, "just as health is the manifestation of holiness. Sickness and health are not simply physical states. . . . They are rooted in the deepest and most mysterious strata of Being." He introduces these ideas in the context of his views on the connection between religion, magic, and medicine. "In our society," he observes, "the commonality of religion, magic, and medicine is obscured. Our medical doctors have narrowed their view to pay attention only to the physical body and the material aspects of illness. As a result . . . they do not see or integrate the nonphysical forces that animate and direct the physical body," and they do not realize that "health and illness are particular manifestations of good and evil, requiring all the help of religion and philosophy to understand and all the techniques of magic to manipulate. Science and intellect can show us mechanisms and details of physical reality—and that knowledge is surely of value—but they cannot unveil the deep mysteries. You cannot restore health in yourself or in others until you know in your heart what health is."

Lest we despair of ever knowing in our heart what health is, Weil unveils the mystery: "Health is wholeness-wholeness in its most profound sense, with nothing left out and everything in just the right order to manifest the mystery of balance. Far from being simply the absence of disease, health is a dynamic and harmonious equilibrium of all the elements and forces making up and surrounding a human being." Health, it seems, is a mystery explained by another mysterious principle. This is the "mystery of balance."

Weil follows this revelation with an additional "ten principles of health and illness," the most mysterious of which is the last: "Proper breathing is a key to good health." He explains that breathing, since it can be voluntary or involuntary, is a "bridge between the conscious and unconscious minds as well as between mind and body. Proper breathing nourishes the central nervous system, establishes a harmonious pattern for other bodily rhythms, and also regulates moods and emotions. . . . Improper breathing is a common cause of ill health. By decreasing general vitality, it increases susceptibility to agents of disease. It can also directly cause problems in many different systems of the body. Learning how to breathe and working consciously with breath is a simple, safe, effective, and inexpensive way to promote good health of mind and body."

"Breathing" is an important and recurring theme in Weil's prescriptions for health and healing, and it holds a prominent place in *Eight Weeks to Optimum Health*, which appeared in 1997. As far as I can see, his opinions on this subject are largely nonsense. There is not the slightest medical evidence that "improper breathing is a common cause of ill health." All the clinical and physiological evidence points to exactly the reverse relationship. It suggests that many types of disease and physiological dysfunction can affect breathing. Sometimes this secondary change in breathing can be serious enough to change the normal intake of oxygen or the normal elimination of carbon dioxide in ways that further impair health; but the primary causes of the problem are the diseases or the physiological disturbances that cause the abnormal pattern of breathing, not the breathing itself.

While it is true that conscious attention to breathing can help individuals to relax, there is no evidence that the breathing exercises Weil advocates have any special advantage over any other techniques for relaxation, or that they have any special therapeutic powers. Like so many of his other pronouncements, Weil's claims about breathing come ex cathedra from his own self-asserted authority as guru and healer. Much of what he has to say about health and healing in this book and in his later works is just like this fanciful section on breathing—a bald assertion without any credible rationale or supporting objective evidence.

Then there is Weil's typically ambiguous assessment of conventional, or allopathic, medicine. First he concedes that it is not all bad, and that "regular medicine is the most effective system I know for dealing with many common and serious problems," among them acute medical and surgical emergencies. But then he adds that "regular medicine is on very shaky ground" in dealing with other common problems. "I would look elsewhere than conventional medicine for help if I contracted a severe viral disease like hepatitis or polio, or a metabolic disease like diabetes. I would not seek allopathic treatment for cancer, except for a few varieties, or for such chronic ailments as arthritis, asthma, hypertension (high blood pressure), multiple sclerosis, or for many other chronic diseases. . . ." This is a startling list of major diseases to be ruled off-limits for conventional medicine. One wonders which of the remaining chronic diseases Weil is willing to concede to the allopaths, and how he knows where to draw the line.

Some of Weil's criticisms of medical practitioners in this and other books are nonetheless valid. I agree with him that conventional physicians are often too interested in the disease and not enough interested in the patient; too inclined to use expensive technology and potent pharmaceuticals when simpler and more conservative approaches would work at least as well. And he is correct in noting that mainstream medicine, despite its many successes, still has only a limited ability to change the course of many serious chronic illnesses. Yet that hardly justifies Weil's sweeping and irresponsible dismissal of allopathic medicine's role in the diagnosis, the management, and the palliation of all the serious illnesses that he enumerates and the indeterminate list to which he alludes. He implies that alternative medicine could do better, but there is no published evidence to support that opinion.

And even if Weil's assertions about the superiority of alternative methods for the treatment of some diseases were correct, how could patients be expected to know when to seek help from alternative healers unless they knew in advance what was wrong with them? One of the main reasons to consult a physician is to determine whether symptoms need to be taken seriously and what might be causing them. Weil's advice could result in dangerous delays in the diagnosis and the treatment of serious illness, unless he were also to recommend that patients first seek competent medical evaluation and advice before considering unconventional treatments. That may be what he had in mind in recently establishing an "integrative medicine" clinic at the University of Arizona, in which allopathic physicians prescribe both conventional and unconventional treatments. Still, without credible evidence that unconventional treatments are equivalent to, or better than, standard medical care, even that eclectic approach is seriously flawed.

III

One of Weil's central themes in Health and Healing, and in his subsequent work, is his criticism of mainstream medicine's reliance on pharmaceuticals instead of herbal medicines. The latter are presently enjoying a great resurgence in popularity, due largely to the endorsement of prominent advocates such as Weil, and to the promotional activities of a "natural products" industry that received a big boost in 1994, when Congress gave the industry permission to market herbal preparations with less rigorous oversight by the FDA than the agency exercises over drugs. Manufacturers of herbal preparations can avoid many of the customary rigors of FDA drug regulation simply by labeling these products "dietary supplements." In 1997, the herbal medicine market had sales of nearly $4 billion, and a stroll down the aisles of almost any supermarket or chain drugstore will confirm that business is booming. A cover story in Time magazine a few weeks ago was all about this burgeoning new herbal remedy business and the popular craze for "natural" medicines.

Weil's preference for herbs and his dislike of synthetic pharmaceutical products probably stem from his earlier training in botany and his long interest in the psychedelic properties of plants. It also reflects his belief in the virtues of "natural" healing methods that patients themselves can employ without recourse to physicians or expensive medical technology. Herbs can be purchased without prescription and are relatively inexpensive in comparison with prescription drugs. In earlier times herbs were the only medicinal remedies available, and botany was a part of the medical school curriculum. But then scientists learned how to extract and synthesize the active constituents of medicinal herbs, and medical botany was replaced by modem pharmacology.

Modern pharmacological science now provides physicians with a vast armamentarium of clinically effective synthetic compounds, many derived from or closely related to substances found in nature, others created in the laboratory. These pure compounds can be standardized and tested for purity, clinical potency, and safety far more easily than the complex and highly variable natural plant materials doctors formerly prescribed. In some advanced Western countries—in Germany, for example—herbal medicines are still widely prescribed, but the manufacture, the purity, and the potency of these preparations are far more carefully regulated by the government than in the United States.

Weil doesn't like the modern pharmaceutical industry and he wants us to return to our former dependence on herbs. His arguments are on balance unconvincing, but they are not without some reason. Weil has an arguable case, I think, when he criticizes the pharmaceutical industry for promoting expensive new drugs that have little or no advantage over older and less expensive drugs, and for sometimes being insufficiently attentive to their risks. I also have some sympathy with his criticism of the excessive prescribing of potent pharmaceuticals by physicians, and the common practice of prescribing many drugs simultaneously without sufficient attention to their toxic or interactive effects. There is no doubt that improper use of pharmaceuticals, including mistakes in dosage and even inadvertent administration of the wrong drug, causes many serious mishaps in hospital and office practice. Even the proper use of drugs can sometimes cause fatal reactions. Misuse of antibiotics can cause the development of drug-resistant strains of bacteria.

Still, the fact remains that pharmaceuticals are an essential part of medical practice. Without them there would be no effective treatment or palliation of many serious diseases. On balance, the good done by modern pharmaceuticals far outweighs the harm, though zealous advocates of "natural" remedies (Weil among them) insist otherwise. Even in Germany, where botanical medicines are widely used by allopathic physicians, pharmaceutical drugs are the mainstay of treatment for serious illnesses.

Weil claims that the presence of many different active and inactive ingredients, known and unknown, makes natural botanical products safer and more effective than synthetic pharmaceuticals. This is mostly speculation, since there have been very few clinical trials directly comparing herbs with pharmaceuticals in the treatment of specific ailments. What Weil does not mention, here or elsewhere in his books, are the problems created by the lack of purity and standardization of herbal products. A recent issue of the New England Journal of Medicine contained several reports of serious clinical complications resulting from adulterants or contaminants in commercial preparations of herbs. As an accompanying editorial in the Journal noted, there can be no safe and rational use of herbal medicines without regulation of their purity and their potency—even assuming that there were evidence of potentially useful clinical effects.

Weil has a good word to say for almost all alternative healing methods, except for some practices used by so-called holistic physicians. "Holistic medicine" is an outdated term that formerly referred to many of the same methods in common use by today's alternative healers, but also included other less widely used methods of diagnosis and treatment that have not attracted much attention recently. Why Weil singles the latter out for disapproval is not entirely clear, since his criticisms would seem to apply equally to many of the alternative methods that he does endorse. In any case, after a general review of the latter, he concludes that the belief of the healer and the patient in the effectiveness of the various forms of alternative treatment is the common explanation that ties them all together. This is his conclusion: "Since belief alone can elicit healing, the occasional success of treatments based on absurd theories is not mysterious."

Weil next considers the healing power of the placebo effect, by which he means the faith of the patient and the practitioner in the therapeutic value of whatever treatment is being used. He says that all treatments depend more or less on this faith, and that is why any treatment, real or imaginary, may be able to cure any disease in certain patients by helping them to mobilize their innate healing powers. Sometimes the result is mainly due to the direct physical action of the treatment and sometimes it is mainly due to the patient's own belief in the treatment, and sometimes it appears to be a combination of effects. Weil probably believes that herbal remedies, diet, physical exercise, and other lifestyle changes belong mainly in the first category. Faith healing, therapeutic touch, magnetism, and most of the other more esoteric alternative healing methods would probably be placed in the second category. Meditation, breathing exercises, biofeedback, acupuncture, musculoskeletal manipulations, and yoga would probably be placed in the third category.

How does Weil know that any of these alternative methods, or any combination of them, regardless of the way they work, can cure disease? Because he has been told about, or thinks that he has seen, apparent cures of supposedly incurable diseases that could not be otherwise explained. And where is the documented, objective evidence of such cures? There isn't any. We simply must trust Weil's opinion, and the belief of those who report these events to him. Weil's books are full of such stories, none supported by anything resembling scientific evidence.

Here are some examples. In *Eight Weeks to Optimum Health*, Weil tells about a letter he received from a patient who wrote: "Six years ago (I'm now twenty-seven) the doctors threw the ugly 'C-word' at me and made it sound like a death sentence. (It was bone cancer.) They decided that they were the authorities and I was the victim and the only way was their way, I walked out of their offices never to return. I took up biking (about five hundred miles a week) and running (about sixty miles a week), and ate fresh fruit, juices, and whole grains . . . nothing else. Too bad more people out there won't acknowledge what a little self-determination and using one's subconscious can do to return a person to wholeness." The patient goes on to say that he or she is now entirely well and hopes to "work toward developing programs for others to offer them alternative pathways toward health and wholeness." How do we know that this person really had "bone cancer" and what really happened? We don't know, of course, but that doesn't seem to concern Weil, who cites the case without further comment as evidence of self-induced healing of a serious disease.

In the same book, Weil tells about a woman patient who had "an unusual form of Parkinson's disease" which caused her to have frequent seizures during sleep. Presumably in response to Weil's advice, she tried "acupuncture, yoga, massage, meditation and other stress-reduction work," and finally "respiratory biofeedback," which eventually caused the seizures to stop. Here again, there is no medical documentation of the diagnosis or the alleged effects of the alternative treatments.

A final example comes from *Spontaneous Healing* (1995). It concerns a man with scleroderma (a usually progressive and fatal disease of the skin and internal organs, thought to be an autoimmune disorder) who cured himself with vinegar, lemons, aloe vera juice and vitamin E. How does Weil know this really happened? Apparently, the patient told him so.

it was only a testimonial but, as Weil explains in *Spontaneous Healing*, he finds these stories meaningful. "I collect this material, save it, and take it seriously. In its totality and range and abundance it makes one powerful point: People can get better . . . from all sorts of conditions or diseases, even very severe ones of long duration."

That people usually "get better," that most relatively minor diseases heal spontaneously or seem to improve with simple common remedies, is hardly news. Every physician, indeed every grandmother, knows that. Yet before we accept Weil's contention that serious illnesses such as "bone cancer," "Parkinson's disease," or "scleroderma" are similarly curable, or respond to alternative healing methods, we need at least to have some convincing medical evidence that the patients whom he reports in these testimonials did indeed suffer from these diseases, and that they were really improved or healed. The perplexity is not that Weil is using "anecdotes" as proof, but that we don't know whether the anecdotes are true.

Anecdotal evidence is often used in the conventional medical literature to suggest the effectiveness of treatment that has not yet been tested by formal clinical trials. In fact, much of the mainstream professional literature in medicine consists of case reports—"anecdotes," of a kind. The crucial difference between those case reports and the testimonials that abound in Weil's books (and throughout the literature of alternative medicine) is that the case reports in the mainstream literature are almost always meticulously documented with objective data to establish the diagnosis and to verify what happened, whereas the testimonials cited by alternative medicine practitioners usually are not. Weil almost never gives any objective data to support his claims. Almost everything is simply hearsay and personal opinion.

To the best of my knowledge, Weil himself has published nothing in the peer-reviewed medical literature to document objectively his personal experiences with allegedly cured patients or to verify his claims for the effectiveness of any of the unorthodox remedies he uses. He is not alone in this respect. Few proponents of alternative medicine have so far published clinical reports that would stand the rigorous scientific scrutiny given to studies of traditional medical treatments published in the serious medical journals. Alternative medicine is still a field rich in undocumented claims and anecdotes and relatively lacking in credible scientific reports.

IV

The growing interest of the medical establishment in studying alternative medicine may soon establish the credibility—or the incredibility—of alternative medical notions. In the absence of supporting evidence, however, skepticism is surely in order, particularly since belief in much of what Weil is saying about mind and body, and the ability of consciousness to operate in the physical world, requires a rejection of the fundamental physical laws upon which our current views of nature and the human body are based.

This does not appear to ruffle Weil, who believes that these laws have already been changed. Indeed, he argues that physicians need to understand that modern quantum physics has overturned much of classical physical theory and is revealing a new perspective on nature, in which the observing mind is the primary reality, and can cause natural phenomena to behave oddly. It is time for us to reject the old-fashioned scientific materialism, says Weil. "What most medical doctors do not know is that the scientific model of reality has changed radically since 1900 and no longer views the universe as an orderly mechanism independent of the consciousness observing it."

In one of the final chapters of *Health and Healing*, called "What Doctors Can Learn from Physicists," Weil offers his interpretation of the revelations of quantum physics. Experimental data have shown that when observed one way, light seems to be acting like a wave, and when observed another way, it acts like a stream of particles. Quantum theory embraces that paradox in a probabilistic, mathematical description of subatomic physical phenomena that seems incomprehensible to common sense and ordinary experience, but that accords with the experimental data. Weil's interpretation of quantum theory is that it forces us "to consider consciousness [by which he presumably means the mind of the observer] as an active agent in the formation of reality, inseparable from it." And so he concludes that "in the world of ordinary experience, the materialistic and mechanistic theories of the past may continue to seem right and work as reasonable approximations, but if consciousness has to be included to explain observed properties of atomic particles, it cannot be independent of systems composed of those particles, whether rocks, stars, plants, or, especially, human beings." According to Weil, quantum physics in effect validates his "stoned thinking," because it demonstrates that ultimate reality is in the mind of the observer, and thoughts can make anything happen. Thus Weil can believe in miraculous cures even while claiming to be rational and scientific, because he thinks that quantum theory supports his views.

Yet the leading physicists of our time do not accept such an interpretation of quantum theory. They do not believe quantum theory says anything about the role of human consciousness in the physical world. They see quantum laws as simply a useful mathematical formulation for describing subatomic phenomena that are not adequately handled by classical physical theory, although the latter remains quite satisfactory for the analysis of physical events at the macro-level. Steven Weinberg has observed that "quantum mechanics has been overwhelmingly important to physics, but I cannot find any messages for human life in quantum mechanics that are different in any important way from those of Newtonian physics." And overriding all discussions of the meaning of quantum physics is the fundamental fact that quantum theory, like all other scientific law, is only valid to the extent that it predicts and accords with the evidence provided by observation and objective measurement. Richard Feynman said it quite simply: "Observation is the ultimate and final judge of the truth of an idea." Feynman also pointed out that scientific observations need to be objective, reproducible, and, in a sense, public—that is, available to all interested scientists who wish to check the observations for themselves.

Surely almost all scientists would agree with Feynman that, regardless of what theory of nature we wish to espouse, we cannot escape the obligation to support our claims with objective evidence. All theories must conform to the facts or be discarded. So, if Weil cannot produce credible evidence to validate the miraculous cures that he claims for the healing powers of the mind, and if he does not support with objective data the claims he and others make for the effectiveness of alternative healing methods, he cannot presume to wear the mantle of science, and his appeal to quantum theory cannot help him.

Some apologists for alternative medicine have argued that since their healing methods are based on a "paradigm" different from that of traditional medicine, traditional standards of evidence do not apply. Weil sometimes seems to agree with that view, as when he talks about "stoned thinking" and the "ambivalent" nature of reality, but more recently—as he seeks to integrate alternative with allopathic medicine—he seems to acknowledge the need for objective evidence. This, at least, is how I would interpret one of his most recent and ambitious publishing ventures, the editorship of the new quarterly journal *Integrative Medicine*.

Integrative Medicine describes itself as a "peer-reviewed journal . . . committed to gathering evidence for the safety and efficacy of all approaches to health according to the highest standards of scientific research, while remaining open to new paradigms and honoring the healing power of nature." The Associate Editors and Editorial Board include prominent names in both alternative medicine and allopathic medicine, who presumably support that mission. Yet the first two issues will disappoint those who were looking for original clinical research based on new, objective data. Perhaps subsequent issues will be different, but in any case it is hard to understand the need for Weil's new journal if he truly intends to hold manuscripts to accepted scientific standards: there already exist many leading peer-reviewed medical journals that will review research studies of alternative healing methods on their merits. During the past decade or so, only a few such studies have passed rigorous review and have been published in first-rate journals. Recently, more studies have been published, but very few of them report significant clinical effects. And that is pretty much where matters now stand. Despite much avowed interest in research on alternative medicine and increased investment in support of such research, the evidentiary underpinnings of unconventional healing methods are still largely lacking.

V

Health and Healing, published in 1983, was the last of Weil's comprehensive and broadly conceived commentaries on health and disease. Beginning in 1995, with Natural Health, Natural Medicine, he produced a series of three "how-to" manuals on wellness and self-care, which established his current reputation as the people's doctor and "America's most trusted medical expert." The next was *Spontaneous Healing*, and the third *Eight Weeks to Optimum Health*.

These volumes follow the familiar, commercially tested patterns of health care manuals by offering their readers "proven programs" for achieving health and warding off disease. Advice on nutrition, herbal therapy, lifestyle, and environmental modifications, plus suggestions for psychological selfhelp, are liberally interspersed with anecdotes and testimonials about patients who are alleged to have achieved dramatic— sometimes apparently miraculous—results through the use of the recommended methods. The recommendations range from commonsensical, generally accepted, and medically sound advice on nutrition and modification of lifestyle to odd, almost bizarre recommendations that have nothing more than Weil's confident assurances and putative "experience" to back them up. Statements are usually made about the curative or preventive powers of some food or herb or healing practice, without the citation of any published evidence. Recipes abound, as do step-by-step guides for certain ritualistic health practices. The rituals and meditations contribute a quasi-religiosity to these practices, which undoubtedly enhance their appeal. All of this is pretty familiar stuff in the selfhelp medical literature, but Weil manages to make it dramatic and fresh enough to attract vast numbers of followers.

The most recent of Weil's publications is *Ask Dr. Weil*, a compilation of questions and answers that have appeared on his website. To judge from the range of questions and the confidence with which they are answered, Weil considers himself an authority on almost every field in medicine. Like his previous books, it includes strong, unqualified recommendations for unlikely and totally unproven remedies, such as massive intravenous doses of Vitamin C to hasten the healing of surgical wounds, and homeopathic medicines and hypnotherapy for the treatment of lupus. It also includes perfectly sensible advice about diet, exercise, and stress reduction that would be given by almost any competent medical practitioner and would find abundant support in the standard medical literature.

In addition to his books, other channels for the dissemination of Weil's medical wisdom include audiocassettes and compact discs on such subjects as "Eight Meditations for Optimum Health" and "Sound Body,

Sound Mind: Music for Healing with Andrew Weil, M.D." His influence is also spread through videotapes of lectures and seminars, and appearances on television shows such as "Larry King Live." Even when compared with the ballyhoo surrounding the other icons of alternative medicine, the marketing success of "Andrew Weil, M.D." is extraordinary. To understand it, one has to appreciate the synergistic interaction between the special talents of the man and the current momentum of the alternative medicine movement.

The alternative medicine movement has been around for a long time, but it was eclipsed during most of this century by the success of medical science. Now there is growing public disenchantment with the cost and the impersonality of modem medical care, as well as concern about medical mistakes and the complications and side-effects of pharmaceuticals and other forms of medical treatment. For their part, physicians have allowed the public to perceive them as uninterested in personal problems, as inaccessible to their patients except when carrying out technical procedures and surgical operations. The "doctor knows best" attitude, which dominated patient-doctor relations during most of the century, has in recent decades given way to a more activist, consumer-oriented view of the patient's role. Moreover, many other licensed healthcare professionals, such as nursepractitioners, psychotherapists, pharmacists, and chiropractors, are providing services once exclusively reserved to allopathic physicians.

The net result of all these developments has been a weakening of the hegemony that allopathic medicine once exercised over the health care system, and a growing interest by the public in exploring other healing approaches. The authority of allopathic medicine is also being challenged by a swelling current of mysticism and antiscientism. that runs deep through our culture. Even as the number and the complexity of urgent technological and scientific issues facing contemporary society increase, there seems to be a growing public distrust of the scientific outlook and a reawakening of interest in mysticism and spiritualism.

All this obscurantism has given powerful impetus to the alternative medicine movement, with its emphasis on the power of mind over matter. And so consumer demand for alternative remedies is rising, as is public and private financial support for their study and clinical use. It is no wonder that practicing physicians, the academic medical establishment, and the National Institutes of Health are all finding reasons to pay more attention to the alternative medicine movement Indeed, it is becoming politically incorrect for the movement's critics to express their skepticism too strongly in public.

Weil would seem at first to be ideally suited to be a leader of the alternative medicine movement at this juncture. He is articulate, self-assured, intellectually nimble—and wonderfully ambiguous. Ambiguity, after all, should be helpful to those who would defend systems of healing that are based on irrational or nonexistent theories and are supported by no credible empirical evidence. But Weil wants to do more than to defend and to advocate the use of alternative healing. He wants to reform the medical establishment. His goal, he says, is to change the "paradigm" of medicine by integrating alternative methods and modes of thought into the teachings and practice of mainstream medicine. That is his declared mission at the University of Arizona College of Medicine.

He seems to believe that he is qualified to accomplish this great reform because he has no difficulty in arguing on both sides of the debate between alternative and traditional healing. In an interview he gave last year, when asked whether he sometimes feels torn between his traditional medical training at Harvard and the new alternatives, Weil replied: "I really think I'm in the middle. Sometimes I'm attacking traditional medicine, sometimes I'm defending it; sometimes I'm defending alternative medicine and sometimes attacking it, so I think I'm pretty even-handed in my criticism. I'm unique in that I'm not aligned with any one school of thought." That may be how Weil really thinks about himself and his "integrative" approach, but on close examination his position makes little sense. He cannot have the argument both ways.

As Weil clearly points out in his earlier books, alternative healing is based on a conception of nature and a theory of learning the truth about nature that is fundamentally at odds with the "straight," evidence-based thinking of mainstream medicine. As defined by Well, and by most of the other gurus of alternative medicine, alternative and mainstream medicine are not simply different methods of treating illness. They are basically incompatible views of reality and how the material world works, and they cannot easily be combined into any rational and coherent "integrated" curriculum.

Is there an objective real world out there, of which human bodies are a part? If so, how do we learn about it? How do we determine whether a method of healing is effective or not? Do we follow the universal rule of science, as explained by Feynman, that objective, verifiable observation is the. ultimate and final judge of the truth of an idea, or do we use the subjective methods advocated by the alternative medicine gurus and described by Weil in his "Stonesville" chapter? Without agreement on such basic issues, it is hard to know what Weil means by being "even-handed" in dealing with the two types of medical practice. Sometimes he seems to believe in the primacy of objective evidence and talks like a scientist, but more often he does not. This is inconsistency and confusion, not evenhandedness. It is hardly a useful basis for the "new paradigm" of "integrative medicine" that Well is promoting,

There is no doubt that modem medicine as it is now practiced needs to improve its relations with patients, and that some of the criticisms leveled against it by people such as Weil—and by many more within the medical establishment itself—are valid. There also can be no doubt that a few of the "natural" medicines and healing methods now being used by practitioners of alternative medicine will prove, after testing, to be safe and effective. This, after all, has been the way in which many important therapeutic agents and treatments have found their way into standard medical practice in the past. Mainstream medicine should continue to be open to the testing of selected unconventional treatments. In keeping an open mind, however, the medical establishment in this country must not lose its scientific compass or weaken its commitment to rational thought and the rule of evidence.

There are not two kinds of medicine, one conventional and the other unconventional, that can be practiced jointly in a new kind of "integrative medicine." Nor, as Andrew Weil and his friends also would have us believe, are there two kinds of thinking, or two ways to find out which treatments work and which do not. In the best kind of medical practice, all proposed treatments must be tested objectively. In the end, there will only be treatments that pass that test and those that do not, those that are proven worthwhile and those that are not. Can there be any reasonable "alternative"?

8

NATUROPATHY

Barry L. Beyerstein
and Susan Downie

PEOPLE SEARCHING FOR RESEARCH ON AND BELIEFS COMMON TO NATUR-
opaths will find such material scarce. It is difficult to find methods
that are exclusive to the occupation. Naturopathy is the most eclectic of
"alternative" practices. It changes its methods in response to popular fads
and beliefs. It practices no pool of consistent diagnostic or therapetitic
methods. The most notable things that unite the majority of practitioners
are a penchant for magical thinking, a Nveak grasp of basic science, and
a rejection of scientific biomedicine (which they speak of as "allopathy").

Because naturopathy lacks a coherent theoretical or therapeutic rationale, one has no way of knowing inadvance what one might receive from
a naturopath. One might encounter anything from commonsense lifestyle
advice—eating a healthy diet, rest, exercise, and stress reduction—to an
array of scientifically implausible treatments.[1]

If there is a glue that binds the diverse and changing patchwork of naturopathic practices together, it is espousal of the teachings of the early nineteenth-century romantic movement known as *Naturphilosophie*. The central
tenet of this movement affected the romantic poets and artists of the era and
some noted scientists as well—that there is a single unifying force underlying the entirety of nature, one that steers all of its parts into a harmonious
and indivisible whole.[2] Much like the concept of "Qi" in Chinese philosophy
and medicine, this mystical force is thought to pervade all living things.[3]

A corollary of *Naturphilosophie* is that in order to comprehend nature one must experience it as a whole—i.e., intuitively rather than objectively and analytically. Openness to one's subjective feelings is considered the most reliable means of revealing the workings of the natural world. Not surprisingly, then, naturopathy has been quick to ally itself with the "holistic health" movement. This emphasis on "holism" helps explain an apparent indifference and antipathy naturopaths have demonstrated toward objective, scientific research.

Naturopathy views sickness as a generalized breakdown of the body in response to "unnatural" events in the environment that can he remedied by overall strengthening of the body's resistance. This is in opposition to scientific biomedicine's view that disease is a localized malfunction due to specific pathogens or processes that involve particular organ systems. Biomedicine tailors its treatments to the system and pathologic process concerned, whereas naturopathy claims to "treat the whole person."

Although naturopathy assumes outward trappings and language of science, it exhibits features of pseudoscience.[4] Beneath the surface are magical roots and a quasireligious basis.[5] Healing stems from a supernatural "life force" much like the abandoned principle from prescientific biology known as *elan vitale*.[6] Biologists once believed that this force distinguished living from inanimate matter. It was derived from a cosmos whose natural order was governed by moral laws—as opposed to the inechanistic ones of modern science. For proponents of naturopathy, "natural laws" are not generalizations from observation and experimentation, but rather seem to he the moralistic dictates of an anthropomorphic "Nature"—usually capitalized to emphasize its purposeful, theistic properties. Health is awarded or withdrawn in accordance with one's ability to maintain harmony and balance with the animistic, vital forces of the universe. In committing itself to vitalism, naturopathy puts bodily functions outside the realm of physics, chemistry, and physiology. This is apparent in the following excerpt from the writings of Harvey Diamond, an advocate of the "Natural Hygiene" movement:

> The true case of impaired health lies in our failure to coomply with the laws and requirements of life. All health problems arise from the abuse

of natural laws. . . . Living healthfully is not an art that we must learn,
it is an instinctive way of life to which we must return![7]

LICENSING NATURPATHS

As of 1992, only seven U.S. states (Arizona, Connecticut, Florida, Hawaii,
Nevada, Oregon, and Washington) and the District of Columbia had laws
permitting the practice of naturopathy. According to the home page of the
American Association of Naturopathic Physicians (AANP) on the World
Wide Web, the states of Maine, Utah, and Vermont added themselves to
this list in 1996. California no longer licenses new naturopaths but permits
those who were already in practice in 1964 to continue under a "sunset
clause." Others practice in California under licensure as acupuncturists.
Because most states do not register naturopaths, an accurate estimate of
their numbers is difficult to obtain. The AANP put the total in early 1992
at 1,044, but a spokesperson, replying to queries by Raso in 1994, dropped
the number to "more than 800." The same official indicated that efforts to
gain licensure were underway in an additional 16 states. At the time of this
writing, four of the ten Canadian provinces (British Columbia, Ontario,
Manitoba, and Saskatchewan) license naturopaths and two others (Alberta
and Nova Scotia) have applications pending.

Since both naturopathy and Traditional Chinese (TCM) teach that
"balancing" a mystical force in one's body is the way to health, naturopathy has become more popular along with TCM's rise. TCM is now
taught in most of the nattiropathic colleges we surveyed. In states suchas
California that do not license naturopaths, many evade the restriction by
practicing under acupuncture legislation.

FROM WHERE DID NATUROPATHIC DICTATES ARISE?

Just as naturopathy reflects the nineteenth-century romanticism from
which it sprang, the latter in turn bears the imprint of an older tradition of
the ancient Greek mystery cults and the teachings of the pre-Socratic

philosophers Heraclitus and Parmenedes.[8] Their descendants inspired the "counterculture" of the 1960s and 1970s with its passion for egalitarianism, naturalness, and the primitive, entwined in a narcissism that equates truth with emotion rather than reason.[9] At the same time, the humanistic psychology movement nurtured self-actualization, the wholeness of mind and body, personal responsibility for one's health, and the belief that mental conflict promotes disease. The counterculture's reaction to materialism helped revive naturopathy and other folk practices tinder "holistic health" and the New Age.[10]

This metaphysical outlook places a trust in the fundamental goodness of the natural universe and the belief that we warrant favorable outcomes if we follow our "natural" inclinations. Disease is a form of hubris that descends when one trusts in reason over instincts—one gravitates to healthy choices if one follows one's intuition.

Naturopathy also asserts that a "vital curative force" (which naturopaths confuse with what the Hippocratics called *vis medicatrix naturae*) flows through vaguely conceptualized channels akin to the "meridians" of TCM. Impedence, or "unbalancing" the flow of this force, can cause disease. Therapy therefore consists of restoring normal flow through "balancing," "cleansing," or "detoxifying" the system. Constrictions of the vital flow can arise from such causes as "devitalized foods," psychological strain, "autointoxication" (toxins usually entering the body through the bowel), metabolic imbalances, colon toxicity, nutrient malabsorption, and "liver sluggishness."[11] Germs are seen not as specific disease-causing entities but parasites that attack a weakened body that has fallen into an unbalanced condition. Since naturopaths believe that diseases spring from this common underlying cause, all sickness is within their ability to help.

HOW DO NATUROPATHS DETECT DISEASE?

Naturopathy's "energies" and "vibrations" cannot be detected by scientific instruments. Most naturopaths use unsound diagnostic and therapeutic devices based on these dubious "life forces."[12] (A display of quaint machinery of this sort now resides in a special museum founded by the collector Bob McCoy in Minneapolis.[13]) Naturopaths also defend "applied kinesiology," a pseudoscientific technique for diagnosing "toxicities" by subjectively assessing muscle weaknesses allegedly precipitated by refined sugar, food additives, or fluorescent overhead lighting.[14] An Australian government Committee of Inquiry[15] found that a majority of naturopaths use iridology—a diagnostic technique based on the notion that pathology anywhere in the body signals its presence through signs in the iris of the eye.[16] We also found that most naturopaths, looking for spiritual energies, defend Kirilian photography as a diagnostic tool. This process, which spiritualists have long believed allows the human aura to be photographed, has a simple, normal physical explanation—a coronal discharge is created in the gas molecules surrounding animate or inanimate objects that are placed in a high-intensity electric field. This discharge is recorded by a conventional photographic process and has not been shown to have any diagnostic value, psychologically or medically.[17]

"Radiesthesia" is a form of dowsing. The naturopath passes a pendulum around the patient's body and watches for deviations that pinpoint the site of a problem. One practitioner told us that he likes to use a capsule of an antibiotic as the weight for his pendulum because, being a "bad substance," the antibiotic would "resonate" in proximity to diseased organs. Dowsers and radiesthesiests do not recognize the fact that it is their own unconscious muscle contractions (ideomotor action) that move the pendulum.[18]

HOW DO NATUROPATHS TREAT DISEASE?

Naturopaths state that their remedies are spiritual is well as physical. Trinity School of Natural Health offers a Doctor of Naturopathy degree to anyone with no prerequisites on completion of twelve correspondence modules. As stated in its promotional literature,

> The school makes no apology for its stance on issues of faith, such is the creation and nature of man, the resurrection, eternity, or any other subject which does not lend itself to double-blind studies, scientific duplication or investigation, but are essential to the spiritual aspect of the whole person.

The practices we encountered in our survey of the occupation ranged from the generally supportable to the improbable to the disproved. The list includes: "natural" herbs and nutritional supplements, biofeedback, relaxation techniques, acupuncture, cupping, and moxibustion (also borrowed from TCM),[19] massage, enemas ("high colonics"), water baths ("hydrotherapy"), heat treatments, aromatherapy, fasting ("cleansing"), hypnosis, reflexology, joint manipulation (e.g., "Rolfing"), "realignment" of the cranial bones, zone therapy, positive thinking, bioenegetics, breathwork, exercise, yoga, magnetic healing, homeopathic potions, therapeutic touch, faith healing, copper bracelets for arthritis, and various Ayurvedic and Native-American healing practices. One naturopathy home page we visited on the World Wide Web recommended wearing socks chilled with ice water to "tone up the immune system" and admitted practicing crystal "healing." These treatments and diagnostic aids are ineffective or unproved. Some naturopaths we interviewed laughed at certain items in the list but then embraced others that had even less credibility.

Seattle's Bastyr University is a wholly naturopathic institution that strongly advocates these techniques. Recently, it has begun to offer a certificate in naturopathic medicine that is obtainable with only nine three-day weekends of instruction, followed by a "one-week intensive" in subsequent years.

HISTORY OF THE NATUROPATHY MOVEMENT

Naturopathy claims affinity with Hippocrates and medical pnictices of ancient Egypt. Twentieth-century naturopathy owes an even greater debt to the central European "health-spa" movement of the 1700s and 1800s.[20] For instance, much in present-day "natural healing" can be traced to a Silesian shepherd, Vincenz Pricssnitz (1791–1851). In tending his flocks, Priessnitz observed that injured animals often sought out streams, then later emerged apparently improved. From this he concluded that cold water was nature's panacea. He tested water on himself and his fellow villagers, starting with sprains and bruises, then cholera and diseases of the heart, lungs, kidney, liver, and brain.[21] He pioneered a network of spas throughout Europe that evolved into present variants such as the German therapeutic communities known as the *Kurorte*. Through these institutions a German naturopath (*Heilpraktiker*) can offer a collection of alternative therapies (the *Kur*), following the natural healing philosophy of Priessnitz.[22]

Like their colleagues in North America, Heilpraktikers preach "holism" and oppose target-oriented, pharmacologically active substances. The pleasant, often-rural surroundings of these retreats are in keeping with Priessnitzs belief in the therapeutic benefits of bucolic environments. The ancient fascination with "taking the waters" lives on today, as many spas continue to be situated in scenic settings whose spring waters have been extolled since Roman times, somewhat paradoxically, for both their purity and their mineral contents. Different mineral springs have developed reputations for special efficacy with particular diseases.

At the spas, mineral baths are supplemented by group gymnastics; massage; baths suffused with galvanic electrical fields, herbs, and vitamins; hikes; rest; dietary manipulations; and hot mudpacks. In present-day Germany, the *Kur* movemerit generally promotes itself as a preventive strategy and a rehabilitative therapy that strengthens during a period of recuperation rather than as an antidote to specific diseases.

During the nineteenth century, European hydrotherapy ("the water cure") and *Naturphilosophie* crossed the Atlantic to inspire figures such as Joel Shew and Russell Thacker Trail who opened a hydropathic spa in Lebanon Springs, New York, in 1845. The herbalism extolled by the European imports built on ground prepared by an earlier radical crusade for botanical medicine. It was led by Samuel Thomson, a New Englander with no formal education who taught that since all disease stemmed from loss of bodily heat, the remedy was to restore internal warmth.[23] Thomson claimed this could be accomplished either directly by clearing intestinal "obstructions" so digestion could produce the additional heat, or indirectly by causing perspiration. Thomson's principal ways of achieving this were the strong emetic *lobelia inflata* and red pepper, combined with steam and hot baths. He opposed the use of all mineral substances because, coming from the ground, they were, by definition, deadly. On the other hand, because herbs grow toward the sun, the life-giving source of heat, Thomson argued that they must refresh one's health.

Politically, the followers of Tbomsonism exhibited the mix of populism and anti-intellectualism that still pervades the naturopathic community today. Thomson's mistrust of orthodox credentials was expressed in his analogy: book learning is to common sense as aristocracy is to democracy and as physicians are to folk healers. We now know the ineffectiveness and harmfulness of orthodox therapeutics in the early nineteenth century. The Thomsonians' skepticism and preference for less violent alternatives to the then orthodox practices of bloodletting, blistering, and purging were not entirely unreasonable.

American naturopathy also has native roots in the "hygienic movement" of health reformers such as Sylvester Graham in the 1830s. A Presbyterian minister, Graham preached the gospel of vegetarianism, sexual moderation, abstinence from alcohol, the virtues of fresh air and exercise, and, of course, the water cure.[24] Graham, whose "Graham crackers" began life as the quintessential wholegrain health food, also influenced John Harvey Kellogg, another religiously inspired health reformer who was physician to the Battle Creek Sanitarium founded by the Seventh-Day Adventist prophet, Ellen G. White. There, Kellogg concocted his original cornflakes recipe as a complete vegetarian source of nutrients. During its heyday from 1840 to 1870, hydropathy, as advocated by Kellogg, was practiced at over 200 spas in the United States and supported several publications such as the *Water Cure Journal* and the *Hydropathic Review*.

The American hygiene movement entered one of its periodic downturns upon the death of its charismatic leader Russell Trall in 1877. Hydrotherapy all but disappeared before being rejuvenated in the 1890s by disciples of another European, Sebastian Kneipp. A Bavarian Catholic priest, Kneipp rekindled enthusiasm for the water cure along with a renewed interest in herbalisin and "health foods." He also recommended, quite reasonably, a vigorous outdoor lifestyle. However, he also showed zeal for such "natural" bracers as wearing coarse homespun undergarments, running barefoot on snow, and walking on dewy grass.

American naturopathy as we now know it is largely the culmination of the efforts of Benedict Lust who merged Kneipp's ideology with the American hydrotherapy and natural hygiene movements.[25] Lust was a German immigrant who contracted tuberculosis, returned to Europe, and recovered after being treated by Kneipp. Lust became the great proselytizer for "Kneippism" in the United States where he was commissioned to start schools, societies, magazines, health-food stores, and sanitariums to promote the water cure. Lust purchased the name "naturopathy" from John Scale who had coined the term in 1895 for his own healthcare system. In 1902, the Naturopathic Society of America was founded by Lust in New York City. It was renained the American Naturopathic Association (ANA) in 1919. The ANA hoped to welcome under its umbrella virtually any healer who rejected the tenets of the then emerging field of scientific biomedicine. One of the ANA's publications boasted

> graduates from Nature Cure, Hydrotheripy, Diet, Chiropractic, Osteopathy, Mechanotherapy, Neuropathy, Electropathy, Mental and Suggestive Therapetitics, Phototherapy, Heliotherapy, Phytotherapy, and other rational and progressive schools of Natural healing.[26]

Naturopathy today persists in using such methods despite lack of validating research. A proposal before the California legislature in 1994 recorded the following educational requirements for a proposed bachelor's degree in naturopathy: Out of 1,500 hours of clinical training,

Manual manipulation: 75 hrs.
Physical modalities (not specified): 75 hrs.
Homeopathy: 100 hrs.
Medicines of mineral, animal, botanical origin: 75 hrs.
Biofeedback, electro-ocupuncture, vibration: 16 hrs.
Kinesiology: 75 hrs.
"Suggestion," emotion, mind, spirit: 100 hrs.
Hair, urine, saliva, iris, tongue, face analysis: 67 hrs.

Most of the above are methods known to be ineffective. They include all of the last "analyses," homeopathy, and applied kinesiology. Most medicines of mineral, animal, and botanical classes that are used by naturopaths are of dubious usefulness.

Because Lust lacked the charisma of the founders of the other competing "drugless healing" modalities—namely, Andrew Taylor Still (osteopathy) and Daniel David Palmer (chiropractic)—he was unable to impose a uniform dogma on his followers. Despite a period of rapid growth in the 1920s and 1930s, when twenty-five states licensed its practice, naturopathy began to decline again in the 1940s. The effects of the 1906 decision by the American Medical Association (AMA) to refuse licensure to all but the graduates of colleges acceptable to its Council on Medical Education was finally beginning to take its toll, and the numbers of naturopaths began to dwindle. Upon Lust's death in 1945, the ANA he founded splintered into a half dozen separate organizations. Chiropractic colleges, many of which had until then also offered naturopathic degrees (so-called mixers), largely discontinued the practice, and several competing naturopathic schools sprang up to fill the void, most by offering mail-order degrees. Each grafted onto the virtues of fresh air, unrefined foods, pure water, light, herbs, and exercise its own eccentric health fixations. A number of splinter groups attempted to reverse this downward drift by regrouping to form a united front under the banner of the American Association of Naturopathic Physicians (AANP) in 1956. Despite some successes, progress remained sluggish. This was due in part to the burgeoning public prestige of scientific medicine following its highly visible successes during World War II and the growing hegemony of biomedicine in the governmental, insurance, educational, research, and technological sectors. During the 1950s, the legislative rights won by earlier naturopaths were rapidly eroded. The AMA opposed "drugless healers" and publicized their low educational standards and shaky scientific support.

After the war, legislative restrictions further hampered the growth of naturopathy. Its practice became a gross misdemeanor in the states of Tennessee and Texas. It was declared unconstitutional in California, though the "sunset law" of 1964 permitted existing practitioners to continue. The Pacific Northwest bucked this trend, however, preserving its reputation as a sanctuary for maverick social movements and medical systems. Washington, Oregon, and the Canadian province of British Columbia continued to provide a relatively friendly environment for "sanipracters" as naturopaths began to call themselves. Nonetheless, naturopathy had to await maturation of holdovers from the 1960s counterculture, New Age prophets of "naturalism," anti "holism" to regain its former popularity.

EDUCATION OF NATUROPATHS

The Doctor of Naturopathy (ND) degree is currently offered by three full-time schools of naturopathy in the United States and one in Canada. In 1956 the National College of Naturopathic Medicine (NCNM) was established in Portland, Oregon. A number of smaller institutions and correspondence schools followed, many of them little more than for-profit "diploma mills" (for details, see Baer 1992,[27] or consult the several naturopathy home pages on the World Wide Web). In 1978, three Seattle-based graduates of the NCNM founded the John Bastyr College of Naturopathic Medicine (JBCNM), later to become Bastyr University. Recently, this contingent of four-year noncorrespondence institutions was augmented by the advent of the Southwest College of Naturopathic Medicine and Health Sciences in Scottsdale, Arizona. According to Raso,[28] most of its funding came from companies marketing dietaty supplements, homeopathic remedies, and medicinal herbs. Others, such as Ulett,[29] have questioned the ethics of the relationship between naturopaths and the manufacturers and distributors of these products.

In the late 1970s, JBCNM received its Candidacy for Accreditation by the Northwest Association of Schools and Colleges, a first for any naturopathic institution. In 1987, the U.S. Secretary of Education approved the Council on Naturopathic Medical Education (CNME) as an accrediting board for naturopathic schools. Most education-accrediting panels assess the academic merits of the curriculum and professional competence of faculty. The Department of Education and the accrediting board, however, were and are concerned not with academic merit, but solely with "factors such as record keeping, physical assets, financial status, makeup of the governing body, catalogue characteristics, nondiscrimination policy, and self-evaluation system."[30]

The full-time institutions typically require an undergraduate degree for admission, though nor necessarily in science. Our survey of entrance requirements indicated that the minimutri grade-point average for admission tends to be quite a bit lower than that of most post-baccalaureate programs. The curricula generally include two years of basic sciences, including human anatomy and physiology, and two years of clinical natturopathy. The basic science portions of the required curricula appear acceptable, but our investigations incline us to believe that actual delivery has improved little since the aforementioned Australian Committee of Inquiry issued its findings in 1977. After attending some of these courses in person, this committee concluded:

> Although the Committee found the syllabuses of many [naturopathic] colleges were reasonable in their coverage of basic biomedical sciences on paper, the actual instruction bore little relationship to the [publicized] course. . . . [Lectures were] exposition[s] of the terminology of the medical sciences, at a level of dictionary definitions, without benefit of depth or the understanding of mechanisms or the broader significance of the concepts.[31]

Present published naturopathic curricula list an impressive collection of courses that might be found in standard biomedical training, but our discussions with graduates of these programs have revealed glaring deficiencies in their knowledge of human physiology. This is in keeping with the conclusion of the Australian investigating team, mentioned earlier, who concluded:

> The Committee visited the colleges offering courses in various aspects of naturapathy. In every case, it was considered that the standards in the orthodox biomedical sciences were disappointingly low.[32]

How else could a graduate leave a program seriously believing that there are anatomical connections between the iris of the eye and the liver, spleen, pancreas, and other organs that meter their distress, or that "realigning" the bones of the skull (see below) is either possible or effective?

The catalog of the Canadian College of Naturopathic Medicine also includes such scientifically suspect offerings as homeopathy, hydrotherapy (the "water cure"), and "soft tissue manipulation." One wonders how students at this institution, which requires three terms of college-level chemistry for admission, can fail to balk at homeopathy, whose premises are contradicted by virtually everything they were exposed to in those prerequisite courses. Literature on the Portland-based NCNM's webpage also defends homeopathy, asserting that it "works on a subtle, yet powerful, electromagnetic level . . . to strengthen the body's healing and immune response to provide a lasting cure." "Subtle" in such contexts is a widely used euphemism for "scientifically undetectable." The authors seem oblivious to the harm such a public airing of the college's ignorance of electromagnetism and immunology does to the occupation's scientific pretensions.

The development of naturopathy in Canada largely parallels that in the U.S. Canadian naturopaths depended until 1978 entirely on American schools for their training,[33] and Canadian naturopaths from British Columbia had helped found the American colleges in the Pacific Northwest. The first Canadian naturopathic institution, the Ontario College of Naturopathic Medicine, opened its doors in 1978. It subsequently changed its name to the Canadian College of Naturopathic Medicine. Initially, it required entrants to be already certified in an allied health occupation and taught its curriculum on weekends over a three-year period. A four-year, full-time program was instituted in 1983.

In Canada, a series of federal and provincial fact-finding commissions has recommended against inclusion of naturopathic services in the national medicare system, on the basis that they lack scientific merit and are so loosely defined as to preclude establishment of acceptable standards of practice."[34] It has since come to light that the responses of some naturopaths to questionnaires sent by one of these investigative bodies, the Canadian Royal Commission on Health Services, were "corrected" by officers of the naturopathic association before they were forwarded to the Commission. In addition, when the Canadian Naturopathic Association (CNA) learned that its members could come under personal scrutiny of the Cominission, its then president sent the membership a "checklist" for sanitizing their offices to avoid embitrrassment if the cornmissioncrs canie to call. The letter included the following:

> Does your library look professional? This is most important: these men are book-worms. Dust your books well even if you haven't used them recently. . . . Get rid of all diplomas not directly related to Naturopathic Medicine. . . . The wording on your stationary should be checked. No "quackish" wording or claims must be made; get rid of it at once.[35]

The CNA was also invited to submit a formal brief to the Royal Commission. In their submission, naturopaths supported the establishment of the government.sponsored national health-insurance program but fought for individual "freedom of choice of any recognized, accepted method of treatment." Gort and Coburn characterized the supporting arguments for naturopathy as lacking cogency and pointed out that the CNA failed to satisfy the Commissions request for scientific data to support their practices. Similarly, naturopaths in testimiony before an Ontario government committee disputed the efficacy of polio vaccination and attacked the concept of immunization. The then president of the Ontario Naturopathic Association was questioned about a "radionics machine"[36] that had been seen in his office. He denied that such devices even exist.[37]

The recommendations of the several official Canadian inquests that have looked into naturopathy have all been negative, a conclusion that was reached independently by a similar committee of inquiry struck by the Australian government. On page 99 of its final report, the Australian panel concluded:

> The Committee does not recommend licensing of naturopaths as a vocational group as it considers that such licensing may give a form of official imprimatur to practices which the Committee considers to be unscientific and, at the best, of marginal efficacy.[38]

The committee did recommend official oversight, however, to protect the unsuspecting public from scientifically questionable practitioners. Judging from the experience of one observer, when his wife was treated by an Australian naturopath, the standards of education and care did not improve among Australian NDs after the panel issued this indictment.[39]

For similar reasons, naturopathy was excluded from the Canadian Medicare plan that was instituted in 1965. Instead of embarking on an effort to improve the scientific status of the profession, the Canadian Naturopathic Association opted for an extensive lobbying campaign. Its leadership recommended that members join clubs frequented by members of Parliament, take legislators to dinner, and contribute to their political coffers. At the time of writing, only one Canadian jurisdiction, the province of British Columbia, has partially insured naturopathic services since 1965. We wondered how this had come about.

In our interviews with naturopaths and their associations, we repeatedly asked for scientific justification for their procedures. While none of any substance was forthcoming, many practitioners argued that the fact that the British Columbia Medical Services Plan partially covers their services must mean that the Ministry of Health finds them scientifically acceptable. Deciding to pursue this, we contacted the Ministry in Victoria in Match of 1997. After outlining our request for information, we were told that a qualified spokesperson would return the call, which was done promptly by an official who identified himself but preferred, understandably, to speak off the record. Asked the basis on which the decision was made to extend coverage to some naturopathic treatments, this senior administrator answered that the ruling had been based on political rather than scientific grounds. He said the Ministry was unaware of any scientific research supporting naturopathy. He said that coverage of the services had been extended in response to consumer demand and intensive lobbying by naturopaths. He also hinted that cost-saving had also been a factor because naturopaths are compensated at a lower rate than M.D.s. They siphon off a portion of those with vague, self-defined ailments or chronic conditions who would otherwise congest the medical services sector at a much higher cost per patient.

IS NATUROPATHY A PSEUDOSCIENCE?

Bunge[40] has provided a useful checklist for recognizing pseudosciences. While naturopathy would qualify on almost all of Bunge's criteria, there are a few that are especially noteworthy. They are paraphrased in the numbered statements below.

    1. *Pseudosciences are stagnant, preferring to perpetuate unquestionable dogma from the past rather than progressing as new knowledge emerges from intellectual ferment, debate, internal criticism, and, above all, new research. When ideas do change in pseudosciences, they do so in a cosmetic way and usually in response to popular fashions rather than empirical research.*

In this electronic age, one might expect an organization's page on the World Wide Web to extol its newest theories and latest scientific breakthroughs. Visiting the webpage of the Canadian Naturopathic Education and Research Society, however, we found instead reverence for the past as, for example, in a laudatory obituary for the late Joseph Boucher, ND. Boucher had been a member of the British Columbia Naturopathic governing body and one who helped found the John Bastyr College—in other words, someone who surely would have been on the cutting edge. An internationally acclaimed spokesman for naturopathy, Boucher remained, with approval of the webpage's originators, a strong champion of the eccentric California naturopath, Stanford Claunch, whose ideas date back to the earlier part of the century. Claunch was a founder of "polarity therapy," which claims that numerous diseases result when the alleged left-right electrical polarization of the body becomes disordered. This is treated by the naturopath intuitively "synching" with the patient's "energy field" and laying on of hands to correct the "imbalance." More dangerously, Claunch also advocated "craniosacral therapy," which contends that this energetic imbalance stems from misalignment of the skull bones which must be manually forced back into a healthy configuration. Ninety-five percent of the population allegedly suffers from cranial misalignment. Of course, in the adult, the cranial bones are fused and not "adjustable." Moreover, no competent electrophysiologist has ever detected the electrical fields postulated by Claunch. Undaunted, his supporters still claim that movements of the cranial bones cause movements in the sacrum and vice versa, offering further avenues for therapeutic manipulation. Claunch's other major contribution was his treatise *Exploding the Germ Theory*, an amusing display of biological fancy, again cited with approval on the society's webpage.

After seeking better fare by contacting the Canadian Naturopathic Education and Research Society and the Bastyr University Research Department in person, we had to conclude that research from naturopaths in support of their practices is still a promissory note. They were able to point to virtually none of the core empirical findings, institutionalized review processes, refereed granting procedures, rigorous methodologies, etc., that typify a legitimate scientific enterprise. Naturopaths conduct little research themselves, and when they do, it is generally defective by current scientific standards. Pressed for details of the research mentioned on Bastyr University's webpage, their spokesperson, Carlo Calabrese,

ND, indicated that their primary efforts to date have been surveys of user-satisfaction that employ such subjective yardsticks as patients' self-ratings of their "quality of life." He said a large study is currently under way, surveying a sample of HIV-positive patients who use "alternative" treatments. Since almost all are also receiving conventional biomedical care, and there seemed to be little attempt to control for such confounds, it is unclear how they hope to determine what is responsible for differences in their measures, if any. None of their research has apparently been submitted to peer-reviewed scientific journals.

Concerted efforts to get several other naturopathic associations to steer us to scientific research that supports their premises produced only a handful of references from legitimate journals testing the efficacy of certain herbs. There was nothing to support the associations' eccentric beliefs about nutrition or any of the fringe therapies discussed earlier. The evidence naturopaths themselves presented was almost entirely composed of anecdotes and personal testimonials. In our own search of the relevant scientific literature, we found no compelling support, but we did find other results from empirical evaluations that question the value of the "holistic" approach of naturopathy.[41]

2. *Pseudosciences exhibit a general outlook that countenances immaterial entities and processes and untestable hypotheses that are accepted on authority rather than on the basis of logic and empirical evidence.*

Radionics, polarity therapy, and therapeutic touch are a few of the naturopathic standbys that postulate immaterial "energy" fields that legitimate scientists cannot detect. Homeopathy has been espoused by naturopaths with little to no evidence to back it up. It, too, posits subtle "vibrations" to explain how pure water can "remember" in order to produce the effects of molecules it no longer contains. As we have seen, naturopathy is thoroughly vitalistic, riddled with unique but undetectable forces and concepts of flow and balance that cannot be empirically tested. Naturopathic "mission statements" we encountered repeatedly stressed the "spiritual" nature of healing.

3. *Pseudosciences are isolated from relevant areas of science that they ought to learn from and contribute to. Bogus sciences have little interaction with and are often proud of their isolation from authentic science whose findings bear on their claims. Pseudosciences avoid contact with disciplines with which they ought to interact on a regular basis.*

It is telling that naturopathy has always had to establish its own colleges to teach its philosophy and practices because no reputable institution of higher learning has been willing to issue natumpathic degrees under its auspices. As we have seen, naturopaths; practically never do research that could be accepted by conventional biomedical journals. Nor is the occupation affiliated with any of the academic umbrella groups (such as the American Association for the Advancement of Science, the U.S. National Academy of Sciences, the Learned Societies of Canada, or the British Royal Society) that promote cooperation and sharing of information among specialized disciplines.

4. *Pseudosciences promote hypotheses that are contradicted by an overwhelming body of data from legitimate fields of research.*

The foregoing sections on applied kinesiology, radionics, craniosacral manipulation, homeopathy, etc., are all examples of curricula in naturopathy that promote dogma refuted by scientific research. Similarly, naturopaths, who pride themselves on being specialists in nutrition, are major proponents of unfounded claims propagated by the "health-food" industry. Scientifically trained dietitians have documented the isolation of naturcipathy from mainstream science in this regard.[42] The Australian commission, referred to earlier, found that naturopaths in that country were disseminating potentially dangerous nutritional advice such as the avoidance by children younger than five years old of all sources of protein. Naturopathic publications assert claims such as that "natural" vitamins (e.g., vitamin C from rose hips) will be more beneficial to one's health than the identical molecules synthesized on the chemist's bench. A magical orientation is apparent in the oft-heard slur that manufactured vitamins must be bad because they are derived from "coal tar."[43] This is equivalent to arguing that a house constructed of recycled bricks from a brothel will be inferior to one built of bricks from a demolished church.

If naturopathy is so poorly validated, why would seemingly well-educated therapists and their clients accept such antiscientific approaches to medicine? There are many cognitive biases that can lead both purveyors and purchasers to think that bogus therapiesare beneficial.[44] A historical tradition and habits oftnind have contributed to the will to believe such practices. These include errors of causality and misattribution (thinking a treatment causes improvement because it precedes the improvement), the power of ritual (physical applications, supplement taking), and suggestion.

It is worth noting that surveys show that naturopaths' clientele are above average in earnings, suggesting a relative advantage in education as well.[45,46] In addition, the distribution is skewed in favor of female over male clients.

CONCLUSION

In our inquiry, we provided naturopaths and their professional associations ample opportunity to refute the conclusions of several major commissions of inquiry over the years that deemed their therapeutic rationale lacking in scientific credibility. None of our informants was able to convince us that the field had taken these earlier critiques to heart; in fact, few seemed to recognize that a problem still exists. Throughout, we found underestimation of the power of the placebo. At the sime time, our own bibliographic searches failed to discover any properly controlled clinical trials that supported claims of naturopathy, except in a few limited areas where naturopaths' advice concurs with that of orthodox medical science. Where naturopathy and biomedicine disagree, the evidence is uniformly to the detriment of the former.

We therefore conclude that clients drawn to naturopaths are either unaware of the scientific deficiencies of naturopathic practice or choose to disregard them on ideological grounds. Naturopathy seems to appeal to magical thinking in people with nostalgia for a bygone "Golden Age" of simplicity when things moved at a more leisurely pace—a halcyon world that probably never existed.[47] Despite the scientific shortcomings of the occupation, there continues to be considerable patient-satisfaction among clients. In addition to benefiting from the placebo effect, inatly find their sociopolitical outlook nurtured by naturopaths' antiestablishment, anti-technology stance, and others find reinforcement for their faith in a benevolent, human-centered universe. Naturopaths also attract those who, for one reason or another, have been dissatisfied with their contacts with biomedicine. They appeal to people with illnesses with a strong psy-chosomatic component and those who have chronic conditions for which biomedicine, at present, can offer little. Naturopaths' elaborate history-taking and prolonged "hands-on" interactions provide the human contact and social support that, perhaps unknowingly, many of the so-called worried well are really seeking. They also cater to those with exaggerated fear of side effects of standard biomedical treatments.

To their credit, naturopaths emphasize the benefits of a healthy lifestyle, the value of prevention, and the desirability of using the least intrusive intervention that will do the job. However, their means of achieving these ideals leave much to be desired while fostering scientific illiteracy in the process. Like most pseudoscientific beliefs, naturopathy offers comfort to its adherents. But comfort afforded is not truth implied.

NOTES

1. O'Connor G. Confidence trick. *Medical Journal of Australia.* 1987;147: 456–59.

2. Grove JW The intellectual revolt against science. *Skeptical Inquirer.* 1988;13(1):70-75.

3. "Qi" (pronounced "chee") is the name Chinese philosophy gives to a scientifically undetectable energy that is supposed to permeate all things. Believers in Traditional Chinese Medicine (TCM) assert that imbalances in the flow of Qi are responsible for disease, fatigue, etc. TCM teaches that balance between yin and yang variants of Qi is essential to health. Acupuncture, Chinese herbs, etc., supposedly restore well-being by re-balancing the flow of this spiritual essence. Naturopaths explain what they do by resorting to similar metaphorical usages of the terms "balance," "harmony," and "flow." which in the final analysis boil down to synonyms for "good" and have no meaning in scientific parlance. See Beyerstein B, Sampson W, Traditional medicine and pseudoscience in China (part 1). *Skeptical Inquirer.* 1996; 20(4): 18–26.

4. Bunge M. What is pseudoscience? *Skeptical Inquirer.* 1984; 9(1): 36–46.

5. Raso J. *"Alternative" Healthcare: A Comprehensive Guide.* Amherst, NY. Prometheus Books; 1994.

6. Brandon RN. Holism in philosophy of biology. In: Stalker D, Glymour C, eds. *Examining Holistic Medicine.* Amherst, NY: Prometheus Books; 1985: 127–36.

7. Raso, *"Alternative" Healthcare*, p. 98.

8. Frankel C. The Nature and sources of irrationalism. *Science*. 1973;180: 927–31.

9. Roszak T. *The Making of a Counter-Culture*. New York: Doubleday; 1969.

10. Basil R, ed. *Not Necessarily the New Age*. Amherst, NY: Prometheus Books; 1988. Schulz T, ed. *The Fringes of Reason: A Whole Earth Catalog*. New York: Harmony Books; 1989. Baer HA. The potential rejuvenation of American naturopathy as a con. sequence of the holistic health movement. *Medical Anthropology*. 1992; 13:369–83.

11. Raso, *"Alternative" Healthcare*, p. 102.

12. One that was demonstrated with pride by a prominent British Columbia naturopath whom the senior author debated on TV was a black box with different colored lights that could be shone on samples of hair, sputum, blood, etc. By reading changes in the reflected light that no one but the naturopath could see, he diagnosed the ailments of several donors. The diagnoses turned out to be uniformly wrong.

13. Ver Berkmoes R. Don't touch that dial! *American Medical News*. September 21, 1990.

14. "Applied kinesiology," as promoted by the Biokinesiology Institute of Shady Grove, Oregon, is another pseudoscience that lacks any vestiges of empirical support. It should not be confused with the legitimate science of kinesiology which studies human motor performance by applying the methods of psychology, physiology, biomechanics, and biochemistry.

15. Australian Government Publishing Service. *Report of the Committee of Inquiry into Chiropractic, Osteopathy, Homeopathy, and Naturopathy*. Canberra, Australia; April 1977.

16. Davidson VS. *The Science of Iridiagnosis: Diagnosis from the Eyes*. London: Thorsons Publishers Ltd.; 1951. Worrall RS. Iridology: diagnosis or delusion? In: Stalker D, Glymour C, eds. *Examining Holistic Medicine*. Amherst, NY: Prometheus Books; 1985: 167–81.

17. Singer B. Kirlian photography. In: Abell G, Singer B, eds. *Science and the Paranormal*. New York, NY: Charles Scribner's Sons; 1981: 190–208.

18. Ilyman R. Dowsing. In: Stein G., ed. T*he Encyclopedia of the Paranormal*. Amherst, NY: Prometheus Books; 1996: 222–33.

19. Beyerstein and Sampson, Traditional medicine and pseudoscience in China.

20. Baer, The potential rejuvenation of American naturopathy.

21. Raso, *"Alternative" Healthcare*, p. 100.

22. Matetzki TW. The *Kur* in West Germany asan interface between naturopathic and allopathic ideologies. *Social Science and Medicine*. 1987;24(12): 1061–1068.

23. Starr P. *The Social Transformation of American Medicine*. New York, NY: Basic Books; 1982.

24. Armstrong D., Armstrong EM. *The Great American Medicine Show*. New York, NY: Prentice-Hall., 1991.

25. Baer, The potential rejuvenation of American naturopathy.

26. Quoted in Baer, The potential rejuvenation of American naturopathy, p. 372.

27. Baer, The potential rejuvenat ion of American naturopathy.

28. Raso, *"Alternative" Healthcare*.

29. Ulett GA. *Alternative Medicine or Magical Healing?* St. Louis, MO: Warren 11. Green; 1996.

30. Raso, *"Alternative" Healthcare*, p. 104.

31. Australian Government Publishing Service, *Report of the Committee of Inquiry*, p. 74.

32. Ibid.

33. Gort E,Coburn D. Naturopathy in Canada: changing relationships to medicine, chiropractic and the state. *Social Science and Medicine*. 1988;26(10):1061-1072.

34. Ibid.

35. Letter from the CNA, quoted in ibid., p. 1065.

36. Radionics is the present-day version of the crackpot device concocted by the maverick San Francisco doctor, Albert Abrams, in the early 1900s. Dubbed "dean of the gadget quacks" by the AMA, Abrams amassed a huge fortune leasing diagnostic black boxes. Cracking open one of Abrams's contraptions, his contemporary, the physicist Robert Millikan, described the useless jumble of wires and components as "the kind of device a ten-year-old boy would build to fool an eight-year-old."

37. Gott and Coburn, Naturopathy in Canada.

38. Australian Government Publishing Service, *Report of the Committee of Inquiry*.

39. O'Connor, Confidence trick.

40. Bunge, What is pseudoscience?

41. Bagenal F, Easton DF, Harris E, Chilvers C, McElwain T. Survival of patients with breast cancer attending Bristol Cancer Help Center. *Lancet.* 1990;336:606-610. Southwood TR, Malleson P, Roberts-Thompson P, Mahy M. Unconventional remedies used for patients with juvenile arthritis. *Pediatrics.* 1990;85:150-153.

42. Raso J. *Mystical Diets: Paranormal, Spiritual, and Occult Nutrition Practices.* Amherst, N.Y.: Prometheus Books; 1993. Barrett SJ, Herbert V. *The Vitamin Pushers: How the "Health Food" Industry Is Selling America a Bill of Goods.* Amherst, N.Y.: Prometheus Books; 1993.

43. In magical lore, the principle of "contact magic," or "sympathetic contagion," says that contiguous things acquire each other's good or bad "essence" through mere proximity—it "rubs off," so to speak.

44. Beyerstein BL. Why bogus therapies seem to work. *Skeptical Inquirer.* 1997;21(5):29-34.

45. Gott and Coburn, Naturopathy in Canada.

46. Beyerstein BL. Alternative medicine: where's the evidence? *Canadian Journal of Public Health.* 1997;88(3):149-150.

47. Bettman OL. *The Good Old Days—They Were Terrible!* New York: Random House; 1974.

9

PERCEPTION OF CONVENTIONAL SENSORY CUES AS AN ALTERNATIVE TO THE POSTULATED "HUMAN ENERGY FIELD" OF THERAPEUTIC TOUCH

Rebecca Long, Paul Bernhardt, and William Evans

ABSTRACT

BACKGROUND—THERAPEUTIC TOUCH (TT) PROPONENTS CLAIM THAT humans emit a metaphysical "Human Energy Field" (HEF) that TT practitioners can sense and manipulate via their hands even without direct physical contact between practitioner and patient. As evidence, proponents note that TT practitioners commonly report various tactile sensations as they sweep their hands just above their patients' bodies. An experiment was conducted to determine if, and under what conditions, human subjects could detect via their hands the presence of a nearby human body that they could not see or touch.

Methods—Twenty-six subjects were tested to determine whether or not they could detect the presence of an investigator's unseen hand that was steadied just above one of the subject's hands. Subjects were tested at various distances between hands of subject and investigator and in trials in which various sensory cues were systematically added and removed.

Results—Subjects performed well at 3 inches between hands, offering correct guesses regarding the location of the investigator's unseen hand more than 70 percent of the time. Subjects' abilities remained strong at 4 inches between hands but diminished at 6 inches between hands. Subjects performed no better than chance would predict when body heat was shielded. Subjects who were purposefully miscued by investigators performed significantly worse than subjects who were not miscued.

Conclusions—Participants in Therapeutic Touch sessions may be mistaking conventional sensory cues such as radiated body heat for evidence of a metaphysical phenomenon.

Practitioners of the alternative nursing practice known as Therapeutic Touch (TT) claim that they use their hands to sense and manipulate a metaphysical "Human Energy Field" (HEF) that emanates from their patients. TT practitioners claim that manipulation of the HEF can facilitate physical and psychological healing. Moreover, TT practitioners contend that they can sense and manipulate the HEF without touching their patients. Indeed, TT is typically conducted with the practitioner's hand a few inches from the patient's body.

Despite this lack of direct physical contact between TT practitioners and patients, both practitioners and patients often report feeling sensations of warmth and tingling during TT sessions. TT proponents claim that these sensations stem from perception of a special type of energy that cannot be accounted for by conventional science. These sensations are often adduced by TT proponents as evidence of the efficacy of TT and the validity of its metaphysical constructs. For their part, some skeptics suggest that TT practitioners and patients may be merely imagining the sensations of warmth and tingling that are so often reported in TT testimonials. In this view, TT participants are victims of the power of suggestion and their desire to find corroborating evidence for their metaphysical worldview.

This article reports the results of an experiment designed to address these issues. More specifically, our experiment assessed (1) whether or not human subjects can detect, without using sight or touch, the presence of a human hand when the hand is placed just above the subjects' hands, and (2) the role that conventional sensory cues such as radiated body heat may play in subjects' abilities to detect the presence of a human hand that they cannot see or touch. If subjects are unable to detect the presence of a nearby human hand when all significant sources of conventional sensory cuing have been eliminated, this would constitute evidence against the claim that humans can sense (or manipulate) a metaphysical HEF.

BACKGROUND

TT is today among the most commonly utilized alternative health therapies. TT has enjoyed particular success in the nursing community, where it has been embraced by several mainstream nursing organizations and utilized by nurses in many hospitals in North America and around the world.[1,2] TT enjoys frequent and largely favorable coverage in nursing journals and periodicals.[3]

The success of TT in terms of the number and prestige of its practitioners has drawn the attention of researchers who have attempted to empirically assess the effectiveness of TT, especially in treating stress, pain, and a variety of mood disturbances. Rosa et al. report that 83 research studies that focus at least in part on TT had been published through 1997.[4] As Meehan notes, this research has been inconclusive.[5] The relatively few studies to report positive results for TT have been beset with methodological problems. These problems include the lack of control groups, failure to use blind protocols, the use of only a small number of subjects, and an overreliance on subjects' self-reports regarding the effectiveness of TT interventions. Meehan suggests that much of the TT research conducted to date has done too little to control for possible placebo effects.[6] In a recent meta-analysis, Peters reports that the many methodological limitations of the existing TT research make it difficult or even impossible to say anything conclusively about the effectiveness of TT.[7] Earlier literature reviews, such as a report commissioned by the University of Colorado Health Sciences Center,[8] have also noted similar methodological problems and limitations.

Perhaps in frustration with the great methodological difficulties (and high financial costs) associated with TT research that examines health outcomes, some researchers have moved from attempts to assess TT's therapeutic effectiveness to investigations of the TT practitioner's avowed ability to sense and manipulate the HEF.

Within the theoretical constructs of TT the HEF is a metaphysical manifestation of the flow of vitalistic life energy through the body. Persons who are ill are said to have deficits, blockages, or imbalances in their vital energy flow. TT practitioners claim they can use their hands to detect disturbances in the HEF, correct blockages by "unruffling" the field, and correct imbalances by channeling healing energy.[9] Again, the HEF is said to be sensed and manipulated without physical contact between practitioner and patient. Practitioners typically move their hands over the patient's body at a distance of 2 to 4 inches,[10] although slightly greater distances are cited by some proponents.

Dolores Krieger, one of the cofounders of TT, notes that TT practitioners almost always describe their perceptions of disturbances in the HEF in one of the following six ways: "heat," "cold," "tingling," "pressure," "electric shocks," or "pulsations." The phrase most often used is "temperature differential."[11] TT proponents do not believe that these sensations are responses to ordinary sensory stimuli. Instead, they maintain that TT participants perceive an energy force that scientific instruments cannot detect and that conventional scientific theories cannot explain. For example, Krieger writes that the terms used by TT practitioners to describe the sensations "indicate a common experience for which we do not as yet have an adequately expressive language."[12] According to Krieger, the sensation of heat "is not the sense of heat one feels when a hot stove is touched or a finger is passed through a flame." Rather, Krieger explains, "Therapeutic Touch deals with a very different aspect or conception of temperature differential than the one we currently understand in biophysics."[13]

To determine whether or not TT practitioners can sense an HEF, Rosa et al.[14] designed an experiment in which TT practitioners were asked to detect the presence of an unseen human hand that hovered above one of the practitioner's hands. Subjects and investigators were seated at a table divided by an opaque partition. Subjects placed their hands through holes in the partition. Twenty-one TT practitioners were tested. In 280 trials, these TT practitioners could correctly identify the hand over which an investigator's unseen hand hovered only 44 percent of the time, a rate that is no better than that which would be expected by chance. Ball and Alexander[15] conducted an experiment in which a single blindfolded TT practitioner was asked to detect the presence or absence of a human body that, when present, was positioned (on a massage table) 4 inches from the practitioner's hands. This practitioner was successful in 7 out of 10 trials, a success rate that Ball and Alexander deemed insufficient to warrant concluding that the TT practitioner was able to detect HEFs.

The results reported by Rosa et al.[16] and Ball and Alexander[17] make sense in terms of science. Given what we know about electromagnetic fields and human physiology, it does indeed seem unlikely that HEFs exist and function in the manner that TT proponents believe them to. But science would also suggest that several sensory cues might be readily available to help humans determine when an unseen human body is in very close proximity. For example, radiant body heat might provide a salient sensory cue. Similarly, rustling of clothing or movements of air caused by even the slightest body movements might provide cues that a body is nearby. In this context, it might seem strange to expect that subjects would fail to perform at better-than-chance rates when asked to discern the presence or absence of an unseen but very close human body.

In order to adequately blind a test of whether or not human hands can detect the HEF of a nearby human body, it is necessary to eliminate any conventional sensory stimuli that could either (1) cue the subjects as to the presence of the body, or (2) miscue the subjects. The experimental apparatuses and procedures themselves may introduce confounding sensory cues. Investigator speech and behavior during experimental protocols may introduce them. Cuing often creeps into experimental protocols in the most surprising and sometimes seemingly inexplicable ways.[18] The seeming inevitability of subtle but nonetheless confounding cues such as rustling shirt sleeves and investigator tone of voice have led experimenters in sciences such as medicine, psychology, and sociology to adopt double-blind conditions whenever possible.

We discovered during pilot testing that subjects could seemingly be cued (and miscued) by investigators' body movements. For example, subtle sounds associated with the rustling of clothing or paperwork by the investigator were sufficient to cue some test subjects. In addition, some subjects could detect a very slight flow of air onto the hand if the investigator's hand was placed over it too rapidly or with a downward movement. Curiously, this slight breeze cued some subjects and miscued others who interpreted the sensation as coolness and therefore selected the wrong (i.e., warmer) hand. Similar subtle but significant cuing and miscuing effects were observed with some test subjects when an air conditioning system was running and the placement of the investigator's hand over the subject's hand blocked the flow of air.

Subjects were seemingly cued (and miscued) when the investigator rested an elbow on the experimental table, which turned out to be a common investigator tendency, especially when testing time was lengthy. Subjects displayed an ability to sense the vibrations or slight change in table alignment caused by this practice, and tended to preferentially guess the hand in front of the investigator's elbow. This resulted in both cuing and miscuing because the investigator's elbow was not always in front of the subject's hand over which the investigator's hand was placed.

Subjects were also seemingly cued and miscued when investigators gave a verbal signal (e.g., "okay," "ready") to indicate that their hand was in position. Investigators tended to look at the hand they were holding in place and subjects could seemingly detect the direction from which the audible signal was issued. We found evidence to suggest that investigators could miscue subjects by issuing an audible signal while looking at the wrong hand, as investigators did on occasion.

Rosa et al.[19] asked subjects to place their palms in an upward position, a procedure we adopted (even if the palms-upward position is not typically used in TT practice). However, we discovered that subjects who were asked to keep their palms turned upward often complained of discomfort and reported "tingling," "pulsating," and "electrical" sensations in their hands. Subjects understandably expressed concerns that these sensations might interfere with their ability to detect sensations relevant to the experiment.

In short, there is a danger that experimental designs of this type may introduce sensory cues that threaten the validity of the study. Investigators may intentionally or (more likely) unintentionally introduce confounding sensory cues, and subjects may consciously or unconsciously make use of these cues. Because it is impractical to double-blind such an experiment, it is especially important to rigorously blind the subjects with

respect to the investigator. In designing our experiment, we tried to minimize these threats to validity. We also designed our experiment in part to
assess the potential role of investigator cuing and miscuing in experimental assessments of TT practitioners.

METHODS

Twenty-six subjects were tested under blinded conditions to determine if
they could detect the presence of an investigator's hand that they could
neither see nor touch. Subjects were recruited from among acquaintances
of Rebecca Long (the first author of this report). There were 13 male and
13 female subjects, ranging in age from 10 to 81 years. (A twenty-seventh
subject was tested but his data were excluded from our analysis because
he did not follow the protocol as instructed.) None of the subjects were TT
practitioners, and none had ever been treated by a TT practitioner. None
had more than a superficial familiarity with TT practices and claims.

The experiment utilized an apparatus very similar to that used by
Rosa et al.[20] Subjects were seated at a table and placed their hands
through holes in a large opaque screen. Subjects rested their hands on the
table, palms upward. The position of the screen and the placement of
holes in the screen were informed by the pilot testing discussed above and
designed to minimize physical sensations caused by the awkward hand
position. To further minimize potentially confounding hand sensations,
care was taken to minimize testing time. Subject comfort was verified
before and after each set of experimental trials.

A towel was placed over subjects' forearms to prevent them from
seeing through the holes in the screen. All reflective surfaces visible to
subjects while in place for testing were covered to preclude the possibility
that subjects would receive visual cues via reflected light. No air conditioning or heating system was run while testing was in progress. Room
temperature was 64°F during all trials on one of the two days on which
subjects were tested; it was 74°F during the second day of trials.

Two investigators participated in the experiment. Investigator 1 was
Rebecca Steinbach, an 11-year-old female. Investigator 2 was Rebecca
Long, a female adult. Another person stood nearby to monitor subject and

investigator adherence to experimental protocols and to verify the accuracy of the recorded data. Data were recorded by another participant, who was shielded from view of the subjects and who operated the LED device utilized in the experiment (described below).

Investigators 1 and 2 each tested a different group of 13 subjects, one week apart. Each subject underwent 10 trials in each of the experimental conditions under which he or she was tested. In each trial, an investigator steadied her hand in place over one of the subject's hands. Whether the investigator placed her hand over the subject's left or right hand was determined in advance using a random number table (odd-numbered integers were associated with the subject's right hand and even-numbered integers with the subject's left hand). To avoid creating air movement, the investigator's hand was moved into position over the subject's hand slowly and with a horizontal movement, parallel to the table. Investigators wore clothing that did not rustle. Investigators were not permitted to lean on the table.

To eliminate the possibility of verbal cuing, a red "ready" light was used to signal the subject that the investigator's hand was in place. An LED device was also used to signal the investigator regarding whether to place her hand over the subject's left or right hand. The lights used to signal investigators were enclosed in a box that prevented light leakage that might have cued subjects. Pilot testing confirmed that the LEDs generated no light or heat that was detectable by subjects.

Trials were conducted at each of three different distances between the hands of subjects and investigators: 3, 4, and 6 inches. Hand distances were measured from the center of the subject's palm to the palm of the investigator's hand. A series of colored lines were placed on the investigator's side of the partition to help investigators judge where to place their hands.

In addition to varying the distance between hands, we used two additional experimental manipulations to assess the possible role of conventional sensory cues in subjects' guesses. In one set of trials, the possible role of body heat as a sensory cue was evaluated by interposing a thin piece of glass (from a picture frame) between the hands of subject and investigator. The glass was placed 3 inches above the palm of the subject. The investigator's hand was placed on the surface of the glass.

In a separate set of trials, conducted at a distance of 6 inches between hands, deliberate investigator miscuing was introduced. Instead of using the "ready" light to signal subjects, the investigator spoke the word "okay" while looking in the direction of the incorrect hand. At the same time, the investigator gently rested her elbow on the table in front of the incorrect hand.

Although subjects were given no time limits, all made their guesses rather rapidly, and in all cases the sets of 10 trials were completed in less than one minute per set. After testing, each subject was invited to comment about the trials. These comments were recorded, as were all unsolicited comments made by the subjects during the trials.

RESULTS

Subjects were assessed in six different experimental conditions. Subjects could be expected to make correct guesses 50 percent of the time based on chance alone. Results are reported in table 1, where reported significance levels are based on two-tailed t-tests against the null hypothesis of chance accuracy (5 out of 10 correct guesses).

Subjects performed significantly better than chance would predict at distances of 3 and 4 inches between hands. At 3 inches, subjects tested by Investigator 1 made correct guesses an average of 7.62 times out of 10, with a standard deviation of 1.76 ($t = 5.36$; $df = 12$; $p = .0002$). Subjects tested by Investigator 2 offered correct guesses an average of 7.69 times out of 10, with a standard deviation of 1.32 ($t = 7.38$; $df = 12$; $p < .0001$). Fifteen of the 26 subjects offered at least 8 out of 10 correct guesses. Three subjects scored a perfect 10 out of 10. No subject guessed incorrectly more than 5 times out of 10. One subject who scored 10 out of 10 was retested and proved able to offer correct guesses 30 out of 30 times (these retesting data are not included in our statistical analyses).

At 4 inches between hands, subjects made correct guesses an average of 6.54 times out of 10, with a standard deviation of 1.90 ($t = 6.54$; $df = 12$; $p = .0128$). At this distance, 5 of 13 subjects achieved scores of at least 8 out of 10, and one subject scored 10 out of 10.

At 6 inches between hands, subjects did not perform better than chance would predict, although the results could be interpreted as marginally significant. At this distance, subjects made correct guesses an

SCIENCE MEETS ALTERNATIVE MEDICINE

TABLE 1 : Mean correct subject guesses, by experimental condition

Experimental Condition[a]	Mean Correct Guesses Out of 10	Standard Deviation	t(df)	Significance[b]
3 inches[c]	7.62	1.76	5.36(12)	p = .0002
3 inches[d]	7.69	1.32	7.38(12)	p = .0001
4 inches[c]	6.54	1.90	2.92(12)	p = .0128
6 inches[c]	5.77	1.42	1.95(12)	p = .0751
3 inches, with glass barrier[e]	5.20	1.21	0.64(14)	p = .5314
6 inches, with negative cuing[f]	3.90	1.66	–2.09(9)	p = .0660

[a] Inches refers to distance between hands of subjects and investigator

[b] Based on two-tailed t-test against the null hypothesis of chance accuracy

[c] Investigator 1; 13 subjects

[d] Investigator 2; 13 subjects

[e] Investigators 1 and 2; 15 subjects

[f] Investigator 1; 10 subjects

average of 5.77 times out of 10, with a standard deviation of 1.42 (t = 5.77; df = 12; p = .0751). One subject who scored 8 out of 10 correct guesses at this distance was retested and achieved a total score of 27 out of 30 correct guesses (this was the same subject who scored 30 out of 30 at 3 inches between hands).

When a glass barrier was interposed between the hands of subjects and investigator, subjects performed neither better nor worse than chance would predict, making correct guesses an average of 5.20 times out of 10, with a standard deviation of 1.[21] (t = 0.64; df = 14; p = .5314). Fifteen subjects were tested at 3 inches between hands both with and without the glass barrier. A repeated measures analysis of variance reveals that these subjects were significantly more likely to offer correct guesses when the glass barrier was not in place (F = 26.62; df = 1,14; p < .0001).

When deliberate miscuing was introduced subjects performed neither better or worse than chance would predict, although the results could be interpreted as marginally significant. Subjects made correct guesses only 3.90 times out of ten, with a standard deviation of 1.66 (t = -2.09; df = 9; p = .0660). Again, this condition involved a distance of 6 inches between hands. A repeated analysis of variance measure indicates that there was a significant difference in subjects' abilities to offer correct guesses at 6 inches between the uncued and miscued conditions (F = 9.875; df = 1,9; p = .012). That is, subjects made significantly more successful guesses when deliberate miscuing was absent.

To assess whether or not subjects manifested significantly different results for either one of our two investigators, a between-subjects t-test was conducted on the results obtained at 3 inches between hands (the only distance at which both Investigators 1 and 2 tested subjects). No significant differences were found between results obtained by the two investigators (t = 0.126; df = 24; p < .0001).

To determine if the accuracy of subjects' guesses declined as a function of distance between the hands of subjects and investigators, a regression of accuracy on distance was computed, albeit only for Investigator 1 (who was the only investigator to assess subjects at 3, 4 and 6 inches) and only for her uncued subjects. The resulting equation was:

Accuracy = 9.16 −.58(Distance)

The adjusted R-square coefficient for this equation was .14. This coefficient was statistically significant (t = -2.68; df = 37; p = .01). Accuracy does indeed seem to decrease significantly as distance between the hands of subjects and investigators increases.

We next attempted to determine if this negative relationship between distance and accuracy could be modeled using the inverse-square relationship between distance and intensity manifested in many natural phenomena such as gravity, magnetic flux, and radiant heat transfer. Accordingly, an inverse-square of distance was regressed onto accuracy. The resulting equation was:

Accuracy = 5.15 + 22.15(1/Distance^2)

The adjusted R-square coefficient for this equation was .15. This coefficient was statistically significant (t = 2.83; df = 37; p = .008). This equation would predict that perfect accuracy would be obtained at a distance of 2.14 inches between hands and that near-chance accuracy would result at large distances between hands.

In describing the sensations they felt during the trials, most subjects referred to sensations of heat. In fact, "body heat" was the phrase most commonly used by subjects—both during and after the trials—to refer to their perceptions. Many subjects reported that they made their guesses on the basis of a heat differential they perceived between their hands when the "ready" light signaled them. Two subjects reported "tingling" feelings in their palms, but most subjects identified the sensations as heat.

DISCUSSION

The simplest explanation for our findings is that subjects were using radiant body heat to discern the presence of the investigator's unseen hand. The experimental protocol was designed to eliminate all salient sources of sensory cuing other than body heat. Subjects' abilities to discern the investigator's hand were high when the distance between the hands of subject and investigator was small. Subjects' abilities diminished as the distance was increased. Regression analysis confirmed that subjects' abilities were indeed a function of distance between hands, as would be expected if real energy such as radiant body heat was involved. Subjects performed no better than chance would predict when a piece of glass was interposed between the hands of subject and investigator, a finding that also suggests that body heat was the most salient cue. Finally, in their self-reported accounts of their sensations subjects routinely used the term "body heat" and spoke of discerning heat differentials between their hands when an investigator's hand was in place over one of the subjects hands. Both the trial data and subjects' self-reports are consistent with the explanation that body heat provided a highly salient and effective cue.

Our subjects manifested substantial variation in individual ability to detect the investigator's unseen and untouched hand. Moreover, subjects' scores in the test trials were consistent with their self-reported ability to detect body heat. A number of subjects volunteered that they felt body heat at 3 inches but not at 4 inches. Others stated that they felt body heat at 3 and 4 inches but did not feel body heat at 6 inches. Some reported that they could distinctly feel body heat at 6 inches. No subjects reported that they could feel body heat at 6 inches but not at 4 inches. And in all cases, subjects guessed more accurately in trials in which they professed to feel body heat than in trials in which they offered no such professions.

Our findings regarding investigator cuing suggest that such cuing can influence and even potentially contaminate experimental results. We tested the effects of only two sources of cuing: voice signaling and leaning on the table. Future research would be needed to evaluate the effects of other potential sources of investigator cuing or miscuing.

The results reported here would seem consistent with Ball and Alexander's[21] report in which a single blindfolded subject made correct guesses regarding the presence or absence of a human body in 7 out of 10 attempts. In attempts where a body was present, Ball and Alexander maintained a distance of 4 inches between the body and the subject's hands. The subjects in our experiment made successful guesses an average of 6.54 times out of 10 at a distance of 4 inches between the hands of subject and investigator.

The results reported here are inconsistent with results reported by Rosa et al.,[22] who report that the TT practitioners they tested could not perform at better-than-chance rates when asked to discern the presence of an investigator's hand placed 8 to 10 centimeters (approximately 3 to 4 inches) above one of the subject's hands. Additional research would seem to be required to address these discrepancies and to provide conclusive evidence regarding the abilities of humans to detect nearby but unseen and untouched human bodies.

CONCLUSION

The results of our experiment provide evidence against the claim that humans can perceive (or manipulate) a metaphysical HEF which emanates from the human body. When salient sources of conventional sensory cuing were eliminated, our experimental subjects could not discern the presence of an unseen human hand.

Our experiment has demonstrated that individuals who are untrained in TT can readily discern the presence of an unseen human hand at the distances at which TT is typically practiced (i.e., 3 to 4 inches) when body heat is not shielded. Although TT practitioners may detect an "energy field" of sorts, the most parsimonious explanation is that the "heatlike" sensations perceived by TT practitioners are due to radiant body heat. In addition, our pilot testing suggested conventional explanations for the "tingling," "pulsating," and "electrical" sensations sometimes reported in the TT literature. We found that such sensations may be caused by the hand position used in TT (palms and fingers flattened and stretched), and by the continual back-and-forth movements of the hands. Certainly, our findings suggest that one can readily explain the sensations reported by TT practitioners without recourse to metaphysical theories that invoke unconventional energy fields.

TT proponents may dispute our conclusions because our experimental subjects were not trained TT practitioners. TT proponents may also object that we have not conclusively ruled out the possibility that our subjects were sensing the HEF rather than body heat. Indeed, we do not claim to have definitively falsified the claim that TT practitioners can sense an HEF. However, within the theoretical system of TT, the universal vital energy force of which the HEF is a manifestation is said to transcend matter and to be everywhere. Although glass effectively shields the transmission of radiant body heat, a universal vital energy such as is postulated in TT would presumably penetrate glass just as it penetrates other matter. If the HEF exists and functions as TT proponents claim, then trained TT practitioners should be able to sense the HEF when conventional sensory cues such as body heat have been eliminated. The burden of proof now rests with the practitioners of TT, who must demonstrate an ability to detect the HEF that is distinct from an ability to detect radiant body heat.

Our findings suggest that skeptics should no longer discount the sensory experiences reported in TT testimonials as being merely the products of wishful thinking or autosuggestion. Rather, the implications of these perceived sensations should be accounted for in future TT research. During TT sessions, participants who have embraced TT may fully expect to sense the HEF and its manipulation. The conventional sensory cues that our research suggests are readily available might then provide TT participants with sensations they interpret as "proof" of the efficacy of TT. This process could likely facilitate a placebo effect among TT patients.

Our findings regarding variation in subjects' abilities to sense cues such as body heat also have implications for future research on TT. Perhaps this individual variation accounts for the fact that proponents of TT differ in the hand distances they recommend or utilize for the practice of TT, a fact that has seldom been noted (let alone addressed) in previous research. Researchers should test TT practitioners under conditions (e.g., hand distance) that the TT practitioner feels are optimal. Differences in subjects' abilities to detect sensory cues, and the relationship of this ability to distance, should also be accounted for in designing clinical studies that involve comparisons of treatment and control groups.

Finally, the findings reported here regarding investigator cuing and miscuing clearly indicate that TT researchers must be vigilant in identifying and controlling for potential sources of sensory cuing which could confound test results. This caution would apply not only in tests of subjects' abilities to detect an unseen human body, but also in clinical studies that utilize "sham" TT as a placebo. Confounding sensory cues may be subtle, and they may or may not be consciously generated or interpreted by participants in experimental protocols. Because of the inherent difficulties in double-blinding TT experiments, it is critical to effectively blind the subjects from cuing by the investigators. Future research on TT must control and account for the many, varied, and often subtle sources of cuing.

We applaud the move toward testing the specific claims of alternative medical practitioners. But as with all new research trajectories, researchers (including the authors of this paper) may have only begun to uncover some of the unanticipated difficulties inherent in research designs and protocols such as ours. Still, this difficult work must continue if we hope to obtain solid evidence regarding the efficacy and validity of alternative medical therapies.

The authors thank Jon Cadle, Dale Heatherington, Beth Holley, J. Sandefur, Rebecca Steinbach, and Harry Taylor for their assistance in conducting the experiment. Additional information about the experiment reported here can be found online at http://www.hcrc.org/t-touch/.

NOTES

1. Meehan TC. Therapeutic Touch as a nursing intervention. *J Adv Nurs.* 1998;28:117–125.

2. Rosa L, Rosa E, Sarner L, Barrett S. A close look at Therapeutic Touch. *JAMA*. 1998;279:1005–1010.

3. Meehan, Therapeutic Touch as a nursing intervention.

4. Rosa, Rosa, Sarner, and Barrett, A close look at Therapeutic Touch.

5. Meehan, Therapeutic Touch as a nursing intervention.

6. Ibid.

7. Peters RM. The effectiveness of Therapeutic Touch: a meta-analytic review. *Nurs Sci Q*. 1999;2:52–61.

8. Claman HN, Freeman R, Quissel D, et al. *Report of the Chancellor's Committee on Therapeutic Touch*. Denver, CO: University of Colorado Health Sciences Center; 1994.

9. Krieger D. *The Therapeutic Touch: How to Use Your Hands to Help or Heal*. New York, NY: Prentice Hall; 1992.

10. Rosa, Rosa, Sarner, and Barrett, A close look at Therapeutic Touch.

11. Krieger, *The Therapeutic Touch*.

12. Ibid.

13. Krieger D. *Accepting Your Power to Heal: The Personal Practice of Therapeutic Touch*. Santa Fe, NM: Bear; 1993.

14. Rosa, Rosa, Sarner, and Barrett, A close look at Therapeutic Touch.

15. Ball TS, Alexander DK. Catching up with eighteenth century science in the evaluation of Therapeutic Touch. *Skeptical Enquirer*. 1998;22(4):31–34.

16. Rosa, Rosa, Sarner, and Barrett, A close look at Therapeutic Touch.

17. Ball and Alexander. Catching up with eighteenth century science in the evaluation of Therapeutic Touch.

18. Rosenthal R. *Experimenter Effects in Behavioral Research*. New York, NY: Irvington; 1976.

19. Rosa, Rosa, Sarner, and Barrett, A close look at Therapeutic Touch.

20. Ibid.

21. Ball and Alexander, Catching up with eighteenth century science in the evaluation of Therapeutic Touch.

22. Rosa, Rosa, Sarner, and Barrett, A close look at Therapeutic Touch.

10

THE COLLOIDAL SILVER FRAUD

Rosemary Jacobs

A RGYRIA IS A CONDITION CHARACTERIZED BY GRAY SKIN. IT IS CAUSED BY the ingestion of silver. Unfortunately, I suffer from this condition. There is a whole body of medical literature on it. In 1942, the year that I was born, it was common enough that an article in the *NEJM* stated that every doctor alive had seen cases. Most of those were caused by silver drugs, which like other noxious and ineffective substances, were used by desperate physicians before the introduction of antibiotics.

My condition was caused by nose drops that a doctor in New York prescribed for me about forty years ago. You can find details of my case and references to the medical literature on my webpage: http://home pages.together.net/~rjstan/. If my doctor had read the medical literature instead of the fraudulent ads from drug companies, he never would have prescribed those drops.

In 1995 I went into a bookstore in northern Vermont and looked at a magazine about alternative medicine for animals. I was stunned when colloidal silver hit my eye. It was sprawled in big, black letters at the top of a page appearing to be the title of a whole page "article." My heart started to race. I thought I was going to read about people like myself, gray people. Till then, the only place I had done that was in the medical literature.

To my horror I didn't read about anyone who looks like me in that

181

magazine. What I read was that colloidal silver has been used for thousands of years apparently without any harmful effects on the body and that people with even a trace of silver in their bodies don't get sick! The author claimed that colloidal silver is safe enough to put into the eyes for conjunctivitis and the nose for sinusitis and that it had been used in medicine until 1938 when it became too expensive to produce. She also recommended purifying your drinking water and that of your pets with it. A note at the bottom of the page referred you to her add on another page that advertised the brand that she sold and included her phone number so that you could buy it from her.

Silver in my body has never helped me. I thought a terrible editorial mistake had been made. I wrote the "magazine," but when they refused to print my letter, I realized that they hadn't made a mistake. They had lied to sell the product.

I phoned someone in the FDA who was following the colloidal silver (CSP) scam. She told me about DSHEA, the Dietary Supplement Health and Education Act of 1994. As a result of that law, products labeled as "dietary supplements" can be sold without premarket approval. The FDA cannot do anything until it is proven that a particular product has injured or killed a particular person. Then they can move only against that product, not the ingredient.

I contacted a local reporter. My story became major news in the rural area in which I live. I had never told anyone other than very close friends why I am gray. Everyone must have been wondering. The reporters told me that health food stores sell CSP and that you can also get it through the Internet. You can even buy machines to make it. At this point I wondered if I was the crazy one.

I happened to have a 1975, 5th edition, copy of Goodman & Gilman, the bible of pharmacology, which I pulled. It explicitly states that CSP causes argyria and is ineffective in preventing colds and flu, adding something to the effect that it is fortunate CSP is no longer being used. With a copy of that and some medical articles, I went to a store that the journalists had told me sold the stuff. They had interviewed the owner for their stories. I told the owner that I was discolored by silver in nose drops and that I had never heard of, or experienced, any benefits from ingesting silver. I asked how he knew that the product which he sold was safe and beneficial for something, anything. He said he'd get back to me, and he did. He phoned to tell me that he had the information, but he didn't think it would interest me. I assured him that it would. Actually, he is one of the few promoters who has ever gotten back to me. Most just ignore me and hope I will go away. I suspect that the reason that he didn't do that was that the reporters were on the case and there was a lot of public interest.

When I arrived, he wasn't there. His wife did not appear happy to see me. She grabbed some papers from a shelf behind her, handing them to me to look at, not keep. I asked if I could take them next door to copy. She was very hesitant, but she was also very uncomfortable even though I was being very nice and polite. Reluctantly, she said I could copy the material. It turned out to be a gold mine because, unlike most of the promotional material, it included the dates when the "researchers" published their "articles." These guys weren't contemporary. They were ancient, and all the promoters were quoting them.

I went to the nearest medical history library and pulled the citations then searched for as much information as I could on the subjects. I discovered that the "researcher" mentioned most frequently by promoters, Henry Crookes, an English M.D., was one of the first CSP manufacturers. He wrote papers around 1914 and was called a quack in *JAMA* in 1919. Jim Powell was not a scientist. He was a writer who wrote an article in 1978 on silver in medicine for the now defunct magazine *Science Digest*. Powell's article was called "Our Mightiest Germ Fighter" just like all the present day promoters say. The article declared, "And now it's silver that is finding wholly new uses as a wonder in modern medicine. . . . Perhaps it soon will be recognized as our mightiest germ fighter." The article never mentions CSP. It does describe the approved drug silver sulfadiazine which is applied topically to burn patients. It took me much longer to track down the retired Robert Becker, M.D. Dr. Becker and his books, *The Body Electric* and *Cross Currents* are often referred to as evidence of the safety and efficacy of ingesting silver. Dr. Becker was horrified. He knew what was going on and had been contacting promoters to tell them that he does not think people should ingest silver and that they should not use his name or works to imply otherwise. He gave me a notice that I have posted on my webpage.

For me the saddest of all are the quotes from Robert Hartman's 1939 book, *Colloid Chemistry*, in which the last chapter is devoted to colloids in medicine. It appears as if Hartman was a reputable chemist who wrote a good book up to the last chapter. He got all his information on colloids in medicine from the Henry Crookes Labs and apparently never checked the material with practicing physicians. Promoters today quote p. 536 of his book in which he states that colloidal silver is safe enough to be applied to the eye. Right on the same page it also states that "Intramuscular injections of colloidally suspended lead are of value in arresting certain cancerous growths." Anyone who looked had to have seen it and should have had serious doubts about the reliability of the information on silver just above it.

I wonder now, after all I've seen and heard, how long the collodial silver fraud will continue. And I wonder how many people have been harmed and suffer in silence.

11

MEDICAL CONSPIRACIES AND THE MYTH OF THE "HIDDEN CURE"

Steven Novella

HOW MANY TIMES HAVE YOU HEARD THE RUMOR THAT "THEY HAVE A cure for cancer?" Have you ever wondered who "they" are, or how anyone could be so callous as to suppress a treatment for such a deadly disease, or how vast such a conspiracy of silence would have to be in order to be successful? I hope so!

Conspiracy theories abound in many contexts; they are now a part of American culture. Americans, it seems, have an easy time believing that "the powers that be" are eager and willing to deceive them on a massive scale for a political, military, social, or monetary agenda. After all, some conspiracies are real—Watergate, Iran-Contra, and Abscam just to name a few. It is no wonder that so many Americans believe in a Roswell UFO coverup, that O.J. was framed, and that there is a secret cure for cancer.

CONSPIRACY THEORIES

Conspiracy thinking seems to be a natural part of human behavior, an exercise in which we all engage to some degree. it is easy to speculate about the evolutionary advantages of having an inborn tendency to be on the lookout for potential threats or plots against us. Such tendencies, however, which might be healthy and adaptive in moderation, can be taken to unhealthy and even bizarre extremes.

When discussing conspiracy theories, it is helpful to separate them into two broad categories: petty conspiracies and grand conspiracies. Petty conspiracies, as their name implies, are small, involving a few individuals or organizations. The scope of such conspiracies are likewise narrow and easily defined, and often involve a single event or purpose. No one denies the existence of such conspiracies. They are most likely common within politics, business, and many corners of our society. Whenever two or more people agree to cooperate toward a nefarious end, there is a conspiracy.

Grand conspiracies are another matter entirely. Grand conspiracies involve many individuals working together over many years—even decades or centuries. The scope of such conspiracies is often nothing less than altering the course of human history itself. Individuals who are part of such conspiracies often have high positions in government or other powerful institutions, and may also be members of secret societies. An example of such a grand conspiracy is the Illuminati, who are believed by some to be a society of powerful individuals who have secretly controlled the worlds governments for centuries.

Proponents of one or more grand conspiracies divide the world into three types of people. The first type are the conspirators, those working on the inside, usually with the goal of world domination, or at least the advancement of their social and political agenda. Conspirators are callous, manipulative, powerful, and one might even say evil. They demonstrate almost omniscient knowledge of people and events, and have an incredible ability to manipulate and control events. They are subtle and cunning in their plans and their ability for deception. At the same time, however, they are often characterized as demonstrating extreme naivete and carelessness, for how else would we know about them.

The second type are the saviors, those who see the conspiracy for what it is and are crusading to expose the conspirators and save the world. People who believe in and promote the idea of such conspiracies always see themselves in the role of saviors, They are able to pierce the veil of deception surrounding the conspirators, usually because of unique insight, or a careless and critical error made by the conspirators.

Finally there are the dupes, which are the rest of us—neither involved in nor aware of the conspiracy. We live our lives in content denial of any dark plot to control our world.

The difficulty with grand conspiracy theories is that they tend to collapse under their own weight. In order to maintain the power, influence, and secrecy of such conspiracies, great numbers of individuals must be involved. These individuals must also extend their influence to many seemingly independent organizations and governments. Those who believe in such conspiracies have no evidence that they exist, and blame the conspiracy itself for the lack of evidence. In fact, in a twisted form of logic, they invoke the lack of evidence as evidence for a conspiracy.

CONSPIRACIES AND ALTERNATIVE MEDICINE

Quacks, cranks, and cons of all kinds flourish by exploiting human nature, by knowing what people want and giving it to them. Regardless of the form, medical charlatans all sell hope, albeit a false hope. Some proponents of alternative medicine have been quick to portray themselves as the victims of a malignant "Medical Establishment," their term for the "Big Brother" of medicine who is trying to protect its monopoly by keeping out all the little guys. They play upon people's natural fear of large powerful organizations and distrust of the government, they confuse professionalism with elitism, and then wrap it all up in a compelling conspiracy theory.

For those practicing unconventional treatments, the conspiracy theory also serves well, for it explains why "the establishment" has rejected them and their treatment. Often they do not understand that all scientific endeavors, including the applied science of medicine, advances through self-criticism and a critical analysis of all claims. When their testimonies and anecdotes are not accepted as evidence for the incredible cures they claim, quack practitioners will often invoke the conspiracy as the explanation for their rejection.

Patients, especially those with a disease which is not curable by standard medicine, are eager to believe such conspiracy theories because they offer the hope they crave. It is far better to believe that there is a cure out there for you, with a small but dedicated band of rebels who will defy the establishment to bring it to you (for a fee, of course), than to believe that no cure exists anywhere. No where is this phenomenon more prevalent than with cancer.

The following quotes, taken from a website which promotes the disproven herbal cancer cure of Harry Hoxsey are illustrative:[1]

"In 1924 Harry Hoxsey claimed a cure for cancer, herbal formulas inherited from his greatgrandfather, Thousands of patients swore the treatment cured them. But medical authorities branded Hoxsey the worst quack of the century, and so began a medical war continuing to this day."

"Why won't medical authorities investigate the treatment? Hoxsey charged a 'conspiracy' to suppress alternative therapies. Was Hoxsey a hoax? Or was he 'The Quack Who Cured Cancer?' "

"Hoxsey might save your life, but above all offers hope."

LAETRILE AND OTHER HIDDEN CANCER CURES

In the 1970s a new drug, Laetrile (called amygdalin in the research literature, and vitamin B17 by proponents), was the latest promising treatment for cancer. Clinical trials, however, showed that the drug was not effective, and it was abandoned, like so many dead ends in medicine.[2,3] In 1984, one cancer researcher wrote, "The controversy over Laetrile is nearly at an end, the worthlessness of the drug having been demonstrated beyond reasonable doubt."[4] But that was only the beginning of the story for Laetrile. Once abandoned by scientific, evidence-based medicine, it was picked up by quacks. The Committee for Freedom-of-Choice in Cancer Therapy was formed, and since then they have been holding meetings in church basements where cancer survivors give their testimonials about how they were saved by Laetrile. Of course, those patients who died on Laetrile are not there to give their testimony. Desperate patients, convinced by these testimonials, can then be flown to Mexico where they will receive this miracle cure while their bank accounts are emptied.

Recently Laetrile proponents have been pushing their propaganda very hard. They have published a book, called *World Without Cancer*, which outlines their philosophy. One would assume that such a book, which purports to demonstrate that Laetrile is an effective cure for cancer, would be full of studies and evidence to support this claim. Such evidence is not to be found, however. What can be found is dismissal of negative studies as a conspiracy and in their place anecdotal testimonials are preferred. There is chapter after chapter attempting to make the case for a widespread conspiracy to suppress this new treatment. Their basic premise is that greedy doctors and pharmaceutical companies, who are making billions of dollars on treating cancer, are suppressing any treatments which are too effective so that they can go on making billions of dollars.

Upon examining the hidden cancer cure conspiracy myth, it quickly becomes evident that a widespread "grand" conspiracy would be necessary to actually hide such a cure from the public, and therefore such a conspiracy is inherently implausible. Also, those with the power to commit such a conspiracy are often misidentified and their motives mischaracterized.

The primary flaw in any theory requiring a conspiracy of the medical establishment is the fact that the medical establishment is not one cohesive entity. Certainly it exists as an economic entity, but not, I will argue, as a plausible conspiratorial entity. The health industry consists of physicians, nurses, and other health professionals, insurance companies, private consumer organizations, universities, government agencies (such as the FDA), hospitals, HMOs, and other managedcare organizations, professional organizations (such as the AMA) and pharmaceutical companies and other private industry corporations. Most of these entities are independent and, in fact, are at cross purposes with other facets of the health care industry. Government agencies regulate physicians who are trained at universities, are members of professional organizations, and work for hospitals along side independently trained nurses, for example. Meanwhile, consumer organizations, such as the National Cancer Society, the Multiple Sclerosis society, and others, keep an eye on the whole process and advocate for patients with specific diseases.

Physicians also fill many different roles. Physicians in private practice do make money directly from seeing patients, but there are many physicians who do not. Many work for HMOs or other managedcare organizations and are therefore salaried. Many physicians also decide to follow an academic career and are either salaried by a university and/or make their money from grants for research. For these salaried physicians more patients means only more work, not more money.

Other physicians dedicate their careers to public health, and do not see patients at all. They work either for the government, for private industry, or for professional or consumer organizations. Their primary task is to review public healthcare policy, as well as other policies which may impact public health. They also review and monitor medical practices and conduct epidemiological research into disease incidence, looking for possible contributing or causative factors.

Of these various medical professionals, the ones who would be the first to know about a new cancer cure would be those in academic medicine and research. New potential treatments are first discovered by basic scientists, those who do laboratory research and attempt to discover the underlying mechanisms of disease. The knowledge they discover then suggests possible treatment strategies for those diseases. Drug companies or research institutes, such as the National Institutes of Health (NIH) or the National Cancer Institute (NCI), will then fund clinical research into the potential new treatment to see if it does indeed work, first on animals and then on humans.

The final arbiter of such new treatments is the Food and Drug Administration (FDA). The FDA will review all the clinical research involving one particular treatment for one specific disease and decide if the evidence supports the conclusion that the treatment is safe and effective for that indication.

The private practitioners and the hospitals—the ones who have a theoretical monetary stake in treating patients, are completely outside of the loop. They are the last to know about new treatments.

What about the scientists who make the discovery? If they have data demonstrating a new effective cure for cancer, then by publishing their data they will achieve fame and fortune, literally. Making a major breakthrough like that will make their careers, ensure future grants, get them promoted at the university, probably get them their own lab, and put them in contention for the noble prize for medicine. They will be showered with professional honors and fame, career opportunities, and more money. Even assuming purely selfish and greedy motives for a research scientist who discovers a cure for cancer, they have everything to gain and nothing to lose by going public with the information. The medical school in which they work will also benefit from their windfall.

What about the evil drug companies, though? Won't they simply abandon a new drug that threatens their existing drugs? This argument also does not hold water. Drug companies are always looking for new drugs, because existing drugs have limited patents that run out. Also, any company that patents a new drug which is a cure, or even an effective treatment, for cancer will make billions, even if they lose the sale of existing drugs. Some conspiracy theorists have argued that a particular cancer cure is merely a dietary supplement and cannot be patented by any pharmaceutical company. This would certainly be a scenario in which drug companies can only lose, but for the same reason the drug companies would not be the ones to know about such a cure. If a treatment cannot be patented, then no drug company would be doing research on the treatment in the first place. In order to now invoke a conspiracy, the sphere of influence of one or more drug companies must be expanded considerably, again resulting in an implausible grand conspiracy scenario. Griffin did just this in *World Without Cancer* when he wrote about "The drug cartel's influence over the nation's medical schools; the drug-oriented training given to medical students; and the use of philanthropic foundations to obtain control over educational institutions."[5]

Even if a short-sighted drug company executive decided to suppress a new drug because it was too effective, the scientists involved could still go public with the information, for the general good if for no other reason. Someone of the dozens of people who must be involved is likely to have a conscience. Also, they could eliminate the need for drug company support by applying for a grant to the NIH or NCI. If their new treatment has potential they should get it. Since so much is at stake for their careers, they would be highly motivated to do so. Also, if the treatment truly worked, eventually some other lab, or even some other country, would pick up on it, do the research, and eventually be able to demonstrate to the world that the treatment did in fact cure cancer. This has never been done for Laetrile or any other supposed hidden cancer cure.

Won't such a new and dramatic cure put physicians out of a job, and bankrupt hospitals? Barry Lynes in "The Healing of Cancer," argues:[6]

"A noted cancer specialist in Boston said he believed that if some simple and inexpensive replacement for Chemotherapy for the treatment of cancer were found tomorrow, all US medical schools would teeter on the verge of bankruptcy, so integral a part of their hospital revenues is oncology, the medical specialty of cancer treatment" (Healing of Cancer, pg. 8).

Despite the vague reference to "a noted . . . specialist," could this be true? There are many problems with this argument. The first is that a "simple and inexpensive" replacement for chemotherapy is very unlikely. Cancer is not a single disease, but a category of disease, containing many entities. There is no single treatment which is effective for every cancer. It is therefore very unlikely that any new treatment would be so broadly effective. It is also unlikely that any treatment would be 100 percent effective for every type of cancer in every stage of advancement.

Even if such a miraculous cure could exist, it could not be discovered "tomorrow." Such a cure would have to be tested in every type and stage of cancer, before traditional treatments could be ethically abandoned in its favor. The clinical research to demonstrate such broad efficacy would take many years, giving hospitals and therefore medical schools time to adapt. Physicians and researchers would not be out of work by any such innovation. If the new treatment results in a glut of oncologists, then fewer physicians in training will choose this specialty, and perhaps some practicing oncologists would have to go back to practicing general internal medicine. Some researchers would need to write new grants and change the focus of their research, but they would still have degrees and skills which are of value.

The medical field, in fact, changes all the time. Because standard medicine is based largely upon science and evidence, the practice of medicine is in a constant state of change. New treatments, procedures, and avenues of research are being created as our knowledge expands. At times, entirely new specialties of practice arise. Also, every time a new treatment is discovered, an older treatment becomes obsolete, or at least less important. A new cancer cure, even the maximally disruptive (and unlikely) case of a perfect cure, would speed up this process considerably, but would be nothing new for medicine. The practice of medicine, in short, is not static, it is adaptive.

There is historical precedence for such a case. Earlier this century, tuberculosis (TB) was widespread and incurable. Entire hospitals were dedicated to the chronic care of TB sufferers. When antibiotic treatments for TB were introduced, the chronic care hospitals were emptied and many TB specialists were no longer needed. TB treatments were not suppressed because of the impact they would, and did, have. Instead, the hospitals were converted for different uses, and the specialists changed their practice.

One must also remember that physicians, scientists, and even pharmaceutical company executives are people, with family and loved ones of their own. Cancer is the number two killer in the United States, second only to heart disease. The people involved in any theoretical conspiracy to suppress a cure for cancer are likely themselves to get cancer one day. Certainly, statistics indicate that someone close to them will be a victim of cancer at some time in their lives. It is difficult to imagine anyone so short-sighted, greedy, and evil as to condemn their loved ones, and even potentially themselves, to a premature death from cancer, no matter what the possible gain.

It seems unlikely in the extreme, therefore, that there is a hidden cure for cancer. Such a conspiracy would involve too many individuals; no one would clearly benefit from such a conspiracy; those who are in a position to allegedly benefit are not the ones who would have knowledge of such a cure; and it seems unlikely that anyone would be psychotic enough to believe that suppressing a cure for cancer would be a good idea. Added to this is the absolute lack of any evidence for a hidden cure or a conspiracy to suppress it. Laetrile specifically is a failed treatment that is kept alive only by con-artists, quacks, and misguided crusaders. Despite this, it is likely that the hidden cancer cure myth will survive in popular culture.

NOTES

1. Hoxsey, How healing becomes a crime, http://www. nets. com/hoxsey/, downloaded 3/1999

2. Unproven Methods of Cancer Management, Laetrile; CA: *A Cancer Journal for Clinicians*. 41(3): 187-92,1991

3. Chitais MP, Adwankar MK, Amonker AJ. Studies on high-dose chemotherapy of amygdalin in murine P388 lymphocytic leukemia and P815 mast cell leukemia; *Journal of Cancer Research and Clinical Oncology*. 109(3): 208-9, 1985

4. Nightingale SL. Laetrile: the regulating challenge of an unproven remedy; *Public Health Reports*. 99(4):333-8, 1984

5. Griffin G.E. "World Without Cancer," *American Media*, 1997

6. The Cancer Bureaucracy: How The Real Cures Are Suppressed. *Health Action*, Jan/93; http://www.hans.orgAynes.htm

ETHICS,
FRAUD,
AND
RISKS

12

THE ETHICS OF PROMOTING UNPROVEN TREATMENTS

Lewis Vaughn

ROMANCE IS IN THE AIR. THE MEDIA, THE PUBLIC, THE GURUS, AND THE hucksters have gazed upon acupuncture, homeopathy, chelation therapy, herbal concoctions, magnetic therapy, and any other treatments called "alternative medicine" . . . and have fallen in love. So, as in any romance, current talk about a beloved "alternative" therapy is usually marked by uncritical acceptance, blind commitment, feverish thinking, and occasional cooing.

In this atmosphere, there are two politically incorrect questions that you must never utter: (1) Is this true? (Are there good grounds for believing this claim?) and (2) Is this right? (Is it morally permissible to use or promote this treatment?) We are told that to ask question 1 (and the relevant accompanying questions about evidence and reasons for believing) is to reveal an annoying and pernicious bias in favor of Western science and rational ways of knowing. It is to show a callous disregard for the kind of validation that can come from people's subjective experiences. It is—worst of all—to give offense to those who have strong beliefs about the effectiveness of a treatment.

Fortunately, scientists—being the pigheaded realists that they are—have persisted in asking question 1 and have thus discovered, among other things, that acupuncture is no better than placebo, homeopathy doesn't work, and chelation therapy can kill you.

Question 2, however, is almost never asked. One version of it is particularly rare: Is it ethical to recommend or promote an unproven treatment—one that has little or no scientific evidence supporting its efficacy?

The issue is important because companies, advertisers, special interest groups, magazines, newspapers, television talk-shows, health practitioners, and others often do promote remedies and health practices that are unproven. This practice—for better or worse—can have enormous consequences for all of us.

Most medical scientists and health officials oppose the practice, sometimes warning that there isn't yet enough evidence to recommend a certain treatment to the public. Promoters of unproven treatments strongly disagree and sometimes ridicule officials for being "overly cautious" or "too conservative." Their most plausible arguments usually involve an appeal to the relative costs and benefits of a treatment. "What's the harm?" they may ask. "If the treatment itself is harmless, why shouldn't suffering people be given a chance to try it? There may be no strong evidence that it works, but if it does, the benefits to many people would be substantial. The costs to people—in terms of potential physical harm—are low. So on balance, it's best to urge people to try it; the possible benefits outweigh the possible costs." Promoters may believe that this argument is especially strong if the treatment has some preliminary evidence in its favor or if the monetary outlay for the treatment is low.

But is this really a good argument? Many on both sides in the debate would probably agree that weighing costs and benefits is a valid way to judge the issue. (This approach is based on the fundamental ethical insight that we ought to do what's likely to benefit people and avoid doing what's likely to harm them.) So the question reduces to whether promoting unproven treatments is likely to result in a net benefit to people. Does the promoter's argument show that his promoting leads to such benefit?

Actually, his argument fails. It fails because it's too simplistic, neglecting to take into account important factors in the cost-benefit equation.

One such factor is probability. Few people would judge a treatment solely on the magnitude of its proposed benefit or harm. Most would want to take into account the probability that the proposed effects would happen. Someone may claim that rubbing a stone on your belly will cure cancer. The alleged benefit is enormous—but the likelihood of receiving this benefit is almost nil. If someone wanted to sell you such a "cancer-curing" stone for ten dollars, would you buy it? Probably not. The proposed benefit is great but not likely to happen. The cost, though, is a sure thing: if you want the stone, you'll have to pay the price. So on balance, the likely cost, though small, outweighs the unlikely benefits, though great.

But what's the probability that any unproven remedy will be effective? The evidence relating to the remedy can't tell us; by definition, it's too weak to help us figure probabilities. We can, however, make a reasonable assumption. Scientists know that the chances of new hypotheses being correct are very low simply because it's far easier to be wrong than to be right. For the same reason, the likelihood of new health claims turning out to be true is also low. Historically, most health hypotheses, when adequately tested, have been found to be false. In drug testing, for example, scientists may begin with thousands of substances proposed as medicines, some with preliminary evidence in their favor. In the end, after assessing them all, only a meager handful are proven effective in humans. Some promoters misjudge the cost-benefit of recommending a treatment because they either overestimate the probability of its effectiveness or don't consider the factor at all. They seem to assume that the odds of any proposed remedy being effective are close to 50-50, especially if there's some preliminary evidence in its favor. This assumption is false.

When we plug realistic probabilities into our moral equation, the wisdom of promoting unproven treatments becomes suspect. Even if an unproven treatment has considerable possible benefits, is harmless, and costs little, it may be no bargain. In general, given the realistic probabilities, the most likely prospect is that the treatment will be ineffective. So, in fact, the odds are excellent that people who buy the treatment will waste their time and money. The likely cost outweighs the unlikely benefits. Promoting the treatment is not likely to result in a net benefit for people, but net harm. The possible benefit of a ten-dollar "cancer-fighting" rock may be great, but the low probability of its working makes buying it a bad deal. Promoting it would be unethical.

Clearly, the higher the cost of an unproven treatment, the less likely that promoting it will result in a net benefit. But there's more to the cost of an unproven treatment than many promoters realize. The monetary cost can vary tremendously and may not be low at all. (Many unconventional treatments cost hundreds or even thousands of dollars.) Other costs include the direct physical harm that a treatment can cause (nearly all treatments—drugs, surgery, herbs, vitamins, and others—cause some side effects). There's also an indirect cost: A few people (maybe many people) may take the promoter seriously and stop, postpone, or refuse a proven therapy to try the unproven one—a gamble that sometimes has tragic consequences. Then there's the very real emotional pain that false hope can often bring. In these ways, even a harmless therapy can cause harm. All these costs must be factored into the cost-benefit equation. Usually, they just make the promoter's argument weaker.

But, some will say, what about the placebo effect, the well-documented phenomenon of people tending to feel better after being given a bogus or inactive treatment? If someone who tries an unproven treatment experiences the placebo effect and therefore feels better, doesn't this mean that there is benefit to trying an unproven treatment after all? Doesn't the placebo effect thus change our moral equation?

The placebo effect (which happens in 30 percent or more of cases) would change the equation if it were unequivocally beneficial. But it is not. First, the placebo effect does not happen in every case. In fact, it is probable that in most cases it does not happen. Even when it does, it is often of short duration. So there is no guarantee that anyone will benefit from a placebo in any particular case. Second, placebos can cause adverse side effects (when they do, they're called nocebos). So they're not uniformly helpful. Third, placebo effects can encourage people to continue to use an ineffective treatment when more effective treatments are available. Placebo effects, after all, are not cures, but temporary feel-good phenomena. Fourth, placebo effects often inspire people to promote a remedy to friends and relatives—even though the remedy may be ineffective or harmful. This simply multiplies the problems that accrue to use of placebos. So in the promotion of unproven treatments, the placebo effect is usually not a point in the promoter's favor. Our moral equation still stands—generally against the promotion of meritless remedies.

Now, it's possible that a person could apply the cost-benefit approach in her own life and rightly conclude that she should try an unproven remedy. She could calculate that any possible benefit, though very unlikely, is well worth the cost because no other treatment is possible or because she considers the cost inconsequential. Promoters, however, aren't privy to such personal information about those who try unproven remedies. Promoters can only weigh the probable impact of their actions on other people. If they do so honestly, they'll have to conclude that, generally, promoting unproven treatments does more harm than good.

13

THE ETHICS OF ALTERNATIVE MEDICINE

Lawrence J. Schneiderman

TWO EXEMPLARY PATIENTS

REGINA R. IS A TWELVE-YEAR-OLD GIRL WITH RECENTLY DIAGNOSED insulin-dependent diabetes. Before discharging her from the hospital, her family physician and consulting diabetes specialist try to instruct the girl and her parents in the appropriate program of treatment, including diet, insulin, and regular self-monitoring. However, the parents become upset when they learn what is involved in insulin treatment and inform the family physician they plan to employ the services of an alternative healing clinic which promises to cure their daughter with a combination of herbal potions, macrobiotics, aroma therapy, therapeutic touch, Ayurveda, homeopathy, and guided imagery.

Silas G. is a seventy-two-year old man with Alzheimer's disease. Throughout his slow deterioration to severe dementia, his wife and adult children have consulted numerous alternative practitioners. At various times these practitioners have prescribed herbal potions, macrobiotics, aroma therapy, therapeutic touch, Ayurveda, homeopathy, and guided imagery. When the physician asks the family about these activities, they first are evasive and then respond angrily, "What's wrong with trying these alternative approaches, since the drugs you offer make him sick, and even you admit they won't really help him very much?"

I will explore the general and specific ethical issues raised by these cases for the physician. However, first I will present some background information on alternative medicine.

BACKGROUND

Alternative medicine (also called "complimentary medicine" and "integrative medicine") embraces a copious array of practices, ranging from treatments that are accepted and employed in contemporary Western medicine to treatments that have been condemned as outright quackery. In 1992, a group of leading U.S. practitioners of alternative medicine prepared a report for the National Institutes of Health, classifying their activities into seven major areas:[1]

1. *Mind-body interventions*: psychotherapy, support groups, meditation, imagery, hypnosis, biofeedback, yoga, dance therapy, music therapy, art therapy, and prayer and mental healing.

2. *Bioelectromagnetics applications in medicine*: applications of nonthermal, nonionizing electromagnetic fields for bone repair, nerve stimulation, wound healing, treatment of osteoarthritis, electroacupuncture, tissue regeneration, immune system stimulation, and neuroendocrine modulations.

3. *Alternative systems of medical practice*: home health care, traditional oriental medicine, acupuncture, Ayurveda, homeopathic medicine, anthroposophically extended medicine, naturopathic medicine, environmental medicine, Native American medicine, Latin American community-based practices, and other community-based healing systems.

4. *Manual healing methods*: osteopathic medicine, chiropractic, massage therapy, and biofield therapeutics.

5. *Pharmacological and biological treatments*: antineoplastons, cartilage products, EDTA chelation therapy, immunoaugmentative therapy, and other therapies.

6. *Herbal medicine*: European phytomedicine, Chinese herbal remedies, Ayruvedic herbal medicines, Native American herbal medicine, and others.

7. *Diet and nutrition*: vitamins and nutritional supplements, orthomolecular medicine (megavitamin therapy), Gerson therapy, the Kelley

regimen, the macrobiotic diet, the Livingston/Wheeler regimen, the Wigmore treatment, the Ornish diet, the Pritikin diet, dietary management of food allergies, and the diets of other cultures.

A list of "unorthodox treatments," compiled by the World Health Organization, adds even more to the above, including applied kinesiology, Kirilian photography, impact therapy, reflexology, Rolfing, cymatics, psionics, radiesthesia, radionics, orgone therapy, pyramid therapy, Dianetics, and flower therapy.[2]

Thus, it is evident that an enormous number of activities have been assembled under the category of alternative medicine, and to be fair each one must be evaluated separately. Such a comprehensive task is well beyond the scope of this article.

Although many practices such as acupuncture and homeopathy are known to be widespread in Asia and Europe, it came as a surprise to many United States health professionals to discover how pervasive these and other unconventional treatments have become in this country. Alternative medicine has been called "the largest growth industry in health care today."[3] Surveys suggest at some time or other nearly half Americans employ unconventional treatments and consult some version of alternative practitioners—usually without informing their physicians.[4,5,6]

Recognition of this phenomenon is being expressed in many ways. At least seventy-five U.S. medical schools reportedly are presenting or developing courses on alternative medical practices.[7] Third-party payers, both private and governmental, responding to consumer demand, have already started reimbursing a variety of unconventional treatments including acupuncture, chiropractic and naturopathy sessions.[8,9,10] Interestingly, "HMOs have found that people who utilize such alternatives tend to be healthier than the general run-of-the mill patient and so cost the HMO less. In other words, it is profitable to attract the business of alternative medicine enthusiasts, whether the therapies they receive are truly effective or not."[11]

Many states grant licenses to alternative practitioners, expressly authorize physicians to use alternative treatments, prohibit medical board discipline of physicians using such practices, and mandate insurance coverage. The state of Washington has enacted the broadest legislation. It requires health plan coverage for "every category of healthcare provider to provide health services or care for conditions included in the basic health plan services."[12] Although the statute specifically requires the health service be "cost-effective and clinically efficacious," when insurers attempted to exclude certain unorthodox practitioners on the grounds they did not meet the carrier's standards for provision of cost-effective and clinically efficacious health services, the state insurance commissioner responded by warning that she would "take all enforcement actions necessary" to override their efforts.[13]

It is important to point out that regardless of the popularity of alternative medicine interventions, enthusiastic claims of their efficacy are for the most part seriously out of proportion to supporting empirical data gathered even by advocates. One must look for other reasons to account for their popularity. Even so, it is questionable whether those who are emotionally and financially invested in an unconventional treatment will allow their advocacy to be undermined by data.[14,15] And although "the medical establishment" is roundly criticized for ignoring or even suppressing evidence of the benefits of alternative medicine, the fact is the voluminous studies cited by proponents of some of the best known treatments were conducted without adequate attention to long-established principles of experimental design.[16]

To summarize briefly with respect to a few of the more highly touted forms of alternative practice, carefully conducted reviews of empirical studies reveal no definitive evidence for efficacy in homeopathy,[17] naturopathy[18] and acupuncture.[19,20] In addition, after completing a study of therapeutic touch [TT], an intervention practiced by thousands of healthcare professionals, the researchers concluded that "the claims of TT are groundless and that further professional use is unjustified.[21]

In response to public demand, Congress in 1992 established an Office for the Study of Unconventional Medical Practices, later renamed the Office of Alternative Medicine and then the Office of Complementary and Alternative Medicine at the National Institutes for Health. The disdainful attitude of the Congressional Appropriations Committee toward "the conventional medical community as symbolized by NIH" comes across without much subtlety in the language of the Appropriation Bill:

> The Committee is not satisfied that the conventional medical community as symbolized by NIH has fully explored the potential that exists in

unconventional medical practices. . . . In order to more adequately explore these unconventional medical practices the Committee request that NIH establish within the Office of the Director an office to fully investigate and validate these practices.[22]

Unfortunately, its first consensus report on the efficacy of acupuncture suggests the office may indeed have been more predisposed to validate than evaluate this practice.[23]

The consensus panel concluded that acupuncture, perhaps, was efficacious in preventing postoperative nausea and treating certain forms of chronic musculoskeletal pain—a remarkably muted voice of support considering the vast array of claims on the treatment's behalf. Even so, the panel's limited recommendations seemed to go out of its way to "validate" trials that would not have met the prevailing standards of contemporary Western medical research.[24,25] For example, two favorable reports on nausea prevention cited by the consensus panel are overlapping studies conducted by the same researchers who acknowledge their predisposition to favor the treatment, yet describe blinding measures that are clearly inadequate.[26,27]

This lax level of scrutiny seems to have affected others in the field who profess openminded neutrality. In a mainstream, peer-reviewed article, the director of a Harvard-based Center for Alternative Medicine Research cites only one paper as apparently sufficient confirmation of acupuncture antiemesis.[28] The cited meta-analysis, however, is more cautious, acknowledging that "none of the studies included in this review is methodologically perfect."[29] Dividing forty-two acupuncture antiemesis trials into "good, fair or poor" categories, the review makes apparent even the "good" trials had methodological flaws that rendered them unreliable. As for the treatment's usefulness in treating chronic pain, the most definitive metaanalysis of controlled clinical studies cited by the panel concluded "the quality of even the better studies proved to be mediocre."[30]

It is important to go into these details because many observers have warned that flawed studies tend to overestimate the benefit of treatment.[31,32,33,34] Moreover, since the reported results of all the acupuncture trials range widely, both for and against the treatment's efficacy, they suggest considerable interference by nontreatment factors such as patient-selection biases, lack of blinding, and other confounding factors. Any deviation from the "fundamental principles of clinical science,"[35] makes the outcomes suspect, particularly if they tend to support the predilections of the investigator. As Eddy points out, "pooling large numbers of clinical series will not correct the problem of poor controls, it will only give the appearance of greater confidence, but for the wrong answer."[36]

EVALUATING THE ETHICS OF ALTERNATIVE MEDICINE

Before proceeding to an analysis of the cases presented above, I shall present a general background of ethical considerations.[37] In the United States a few broad principles are acknowledged to underlie medical ethics: autonomy, nonmaleficence, beneficence, and justice.[38]

Autonomy

Autonomy literally means self-governance. In this country, with its long history of tort, battery and informed consent laws, the individual's right to refuse unwanted treatments and participate in personal medical decisions is well established. To serve this goal physicians have the responsibility to make sure the patient is appropriately informed. Thus, it is essential the information conveyed to the patient about offered treatments is accurate and reliable. How accurate and reliable is the information provided by physicians?

Critics claim that a great deal of contemporary Western medical practice lacks empirical validation. (One hears a wide range of percentages extrapolated from limited studies.)[39,40,41,42] Nevertheless, in this and in many other advanced societies, an important development occurred in the last half century: The introduction of randomized control trials to evaluate new medical treatments. Today, we expect claims of therapeutic efficacy to be based on a scientific method that includes randomized assignment of intervention and control subjects, informed consent, clear definitions of interventions and outcome measures, appropriate use of statistical analysis, and confirmation of observations by independent researchers. These are the "evidence-based" standards of contemporary Western medicine.

The goals of medicine have to do with healing (which means to make whole) the patient (which comes from the word to suffer). In other words, restoring health and alleviating suffering by preventing or treating illness constitutes the practice of medicine. Thus any practice—if it calls itself medicine—whether it uses the term, alternative, complementary, or integrated medicine should be expected to adhere to these goals and standards.

We know, of course, there are many ways to fulfill human needs that lie outside the range of medicine. In addition to physical and psychological well-being, we also seek things like love and happiness, spiritual fulfillment, and harmonic balance between labor and leisure. We seek them in many ways—listening to music, praying, working, reading, meditating, hiking in the mountains, being with one's loved ones and friends. These are all ways we seek the good life without claiming that they are part of medicine. They are alternatives to medicine.

Why is this distinction important? It is important because many proponents of alternative medicine do not claim their treatments are alternatives to medicine. Rather, they claim their treatments are medicine. They not only provide such things as spiritual fulfillment, harmonic balance and happiness, but they also cure specific diseases, such as cancer, heart disease, and AIDS.

What can we say about the validity of these claims? I paid a visit to the Alternative Health section of the UCSD Bookstore to see what a few of the most celebrated gurus have to say about AIDS, for example. First I looked in the book *Quantum Healing* by Deepak Chopra, M.D.[43] According to Dr. Chopra AIDS involves a "distortion in the proper sequence of intelligence" in a person's DNA. Siren-like the AIDS virus emits a sound that lures the DNA to its destruction. " 'Hearing' the virus in its vicinity, the DNA mistakes it for a friendly or compatible sound." This is a believable explanation, says Dr. Chopra, "once one realizes that DNA, which the virus is exploiting, is itself a bundle of vibrations." The treatment? Reshape "the proper sequence of sounds using Ayurveda's primordial sounds" which "guides the disrupted DNA into line." "Once the sequence of sound is restored," Dr. Chopra assures us, "the tremendous structural rigidity of the DNA should again protect it from future disruptions." To put it mildly, Dr. Chopra proposes a treatment and prevention program for AIDS that has no supporting empirical data.

Next I looked up what Christine Northrup, M.D. has to say about AIDS in her book *Women's Bodies, Women's Wisdom*.[44] Dr. Northrup contends that the AIDS epidemic is "a consequence of a large-scale breakdown in human immunity, resulting from such factors as pollution of the air and water, soil depletion, poor nutrition, and generations of sexual repression." Her treatment program is vague, flowery and ultimately misleading. "Long-term AIDS survivors," she states, "and those who have reversed their HIV status to negative, all have the same things in common: They have chosen to transform their lives and their immune systems to resume the power of nature and love." Contrary to her statement, there has never been a documented case of reversal of HIV status.

Then I looked in *Spontaneous Healing* by Andrew Weil, M.D.[45] Dr. Weil approvingly presents the treatment plan of a patient, Mark M., who disparages AZT: "All the people I know who used it are dead"—a fallacious post hoc argument that does not require an M.D. degree to recognize. Mark M. attributes his survival to having "a healthy lifestyle and therapies to support the healing system." These therapies include consuming "a lot of raw garlic," hot chile peppers, organic food, "purified" water, and Chinese herbal remedies. In fact, none of these substances and specifically no Chinese herbal remedy, has ever been shown to benefit patients with AIDS. On the contrary, at the time Dr. Weil was endorsing this regimen, a highly touted Chinese herbal remedy, Compound Q,[46] which was being imported and sold as cure for AIDS in underground buyer's clubs, was proving to be highly toxic, producing seizures, and death.

It is particularly dismaying to remind the reader these authors are immensely popular and influential, even respectable—two have lectured at Harvard Medical School and all three have been featured on Public Television. Had they tried to put these statements in a refereed mainstream medical publication, they would have been immediately challenged by their peers. What is your evidence for that? What is the basis for your conclusions? How can you make those factual assertions in the absence of empirical data? And so forth.

These are the kinds of questions that arise from evidence-based contemporary Western medicine. By contrast, much of alternative medicine is sustained only by the authority of theoriespreferably exotic, ancient, and magical. The tradition of Western medicine is quite the opposite: Theories are not inviolable altars of worship but points of departure for empirical studies. Theories are constantly being pummeled, reshaped, sometimes buttressed, more often completely demolished by data. Indeed, to cite an aphorism well known to many a chastened scientist: The Tragedy of Science is when the Beautiful Damsel of Theory is slain by the Dragon of Fact.

Again, we are not talking about living the good life, we are talking about medicine. Medicine cannot fulfill every human need. Yet, with respect to whatever medicine does take responsibility for it owes a scrupulous attention to empirical data. If physicians allow themselves to be uncritically swept up in the wave of enthusiasm for so-called alternative medicine, they risk misinforming and harming their patients. Yes, patients have needs that are not being served by contemporary Western medicine, but these needs do not include being subjected to bogus tests, claims and treatments.

But what about this vaunted principle of autonomy, you might say. If I am a willing patient who consents to treatment by a willing provider, why can't I do that? The answer is, the two of you are (pretty much) free to do whatever you want, but not to call it whatever you want. Society, not to mention the dictionary, imposes certain constraints. You cannot claim, for example, when you consult a tennis instructor to cure your feeble backhand you are obtaining medical care. The tennis instructor might enhance your well-being enormously. Still, neither society nor the dictionary would accept a claim the tennis instructor was practicing medicine. The domain of medicine is (and therefore, alternative medicine should be) defined by certain goals, principles, actions, scope of practice, measures of outcomes, and standards of evidence.

Nonmaleficence

Although the well-known maxim, "First do no harm" is aimed at physicians, in fact it is a general obligation of all members of society. All of us have a general duty to avoid causing harm and, if we are seriously derelict, may be subject to criminal penalties. Nevertheless, nonmaleficence is a particularly important principle in medicine because doctors have such enormous powers to cause harm.

The reader may recall a movie called *Lorenzo's Oil*, which was about a young child with a devastating neurologic disease, adrenoleuko-dystrophy. The movie starred Nick Nolte and Susan Sarandon playing the roles of attractive, All-American parents who had "discovered" a treatment called Lorenzo's Oil. This oil, they were convinced, would cure their child. However, a doctor with a sinister foreign accent (Peter Ustinov) refused to provide this treatment until it had been studied in a randomized clinical trial. The movie was all about the heroic efforts of the parents to go around this obstinate doctor and get their child started on treatment. At the movie's end, the audience was left with the conclusion the parents had triumphed and the child was beginning to undergo a miraculous recovery. Unfortunately, the movie was a fraud. Even by the time the movie had been made, it was clear the oil produced no such miracle. Worse than being merely useless, it was toxic as well.[47,48]

Almost certainly, that movie was designed to exploit the public's perception that contemporary Western medicine is withholding miraculous new treatments from desperate patients simply because the treatments have not gone through the dull routine of clinical testing.[49] This widespread belief is based on a misconception that any new untested treatment is more likely to be beneficial than not. In fact, the odds are quite the reverse. For example, the Pharmaceutical Manufacturers Association estimates for every 5,000 new drugs that are synthesized, 250 make it to animal studies, five make it to human trials and only one gets approved by the FDA.[50] In other words, at each step the vast majority of "promising" new drugs are rejected because they are either useless or harmful. Clearly then, the medical profession behaves irresponsibly if it leads patients to believe the chances are better than even that a new untested drug will be beneficial. Even more irresponsibly, in the case of alternative medicine with the vast array of nonvalidated teas, pastes, tinctures, extracts, enemas, hormones, megavitamin cocktails, and animal skeletal parts that make up its pharmacopoeia, the harms are magnified if they detour a patient away from truly beneficial therapies. This was directly demonstrated in a study of over 500 breast cancer patients which found that "beliefs in the efficacy of alternative treatments including herbal remedies, over-the-counter medications, chiropractic regimens, and, perhaps most importantly, prayer [contrary to those who proclaim its medical benefit] and a reliance on God," substantially contributed to a delayed diagnosis.[51]

Beneficence

Physicians, indeed all healthcare professionals, have a duty not only to avoid harm but also a positive duty to do good—that is, to act on behalf of the patient's best interest. This duty takes precedence over any self-interest. That a number of physicians have violated this principle and favored their own financial interests is no excuse to condemn all of medicine. In fact, when physicians were discovered to be more likely to use services and facilities in which they had a financial interest, it was the medical profession itself that exposed and condemned these actions.[52,53,54,55,56]

Applying the principle of beneficence requires subjecting claims of benefits to empirical evidence, in particular, recognizing the power of the placebo effect. To return to the consensus panel that came out in support of acupuncture for nausea prevention—it acknowledged that benefits were hard to evaluate against the placebo effects of sham acupuncture. Indeed, even in the best studies, placement of the "sham" needle high on the forearm and the "true" placement near the wrist (which caused tingling), made it easy for both the subject and the "neutral" observer to distinguish between the two.[57,58] Therefore it is unlikely the consensus panel had successfully excluded psychological factors that might, by themselves, have accounted for the observed effects.[59] If sticking needles in patients has beneficial effects it would be an interesting observation, of course, but it would also suggest that such accomplishments do not require lengthy acupuncture training or the elaborate theories of a complex meridian system.[60] It is not a new observation that suggestion can achieve powerful effects. In this country and in Europe, hypnosis (our version of acupuncture, perhaps) has been used successfully for over two centuries in a variety of therapeutic circumstances, including to achieve anesthesia during mastectomies and other forms of major surgery.[61]

Another area of alternative medicine in which beneficence has been subverted to profiteering is the rapidly growing business of herbal remedies.[62] Since the passage of the 1994 Dietary Supplement Health and Education Act, manufacturers have been free of the Food and Drug Administration's authority over so-called dietary supplements. As a result, companies can make wide-ranging claims without having to prove efficacy. Although a company cannot claim a herbal supplement cures cancer or relieves depression, it can say that it "promotes prostate health" or "aids in mental focus."[63] In view of this, some critics fear that "pharmaceutical companies will attempt to classify some products as herbal supplements instead of as drugs to skirt the rigorous process required to bring a drug to market."[64] As noted by Dr. David Kessler, the former head of the FDA, "this is not about health and this is not about well-being; this is about money and jumping on a bandwagon."[65]

An objection to the scientific methodology underlying contemporary Western medicine often made by proponents of alternative medicine is in this New Age patients are held to be so unique that no conclusions can be drawn from randomized controlled trials. A randomized controlled trial, they argue, will not tell us that a particular patient will not benefit from homeopathy just because it did not work on 100 other patients. There is a legitimate way to respond to this question. It is called the N of one trial.

I once had a patient, a middle-aged professor, who had just married a younger woman. He began to be concerned about his sexual adequacy and asked me to give him testosterone (this was before the Age of Viagra). From my examination, I regarded him as healthy in all respects and even found that his testosterone level was normal. I was unable to convince him, however, that he was not suffering from testosterone deficiency. So I proposed a trial: For six months I would inject him with either testosterone or saline—he would not know which. We would both keep a record and at the end of six months we would see what the results were. Every month he came in; I filled a syringe with either testosterone or saline and gave it to the nurse who injected him without knowing the contents. As we agreed, I kept a record of the treatment given and he kept a record of his sex life. At the end of the six months when we sat down and talked, he was persuaded by the results that the testosterone made no difference whatsoever. To me, that was an honest use of the placebo effect in a way to help the patient to recognize what was really going on, and it led us to a far more fruitful approach to his concerns. An N of one trial can be used by anyone who objects to performing a randomized controlled trial on large numbers of patients yet seriously wants to examine whether a treatment effect is specific or a placebo.

Justice

The principle of justice addresses the fair distribution of burdens and benefits in society. It is already common knowledge that our country is concerned about the high cost of medical care, the limits of medical resources and access to these resources, in other words, rationing and resource allocation. Although we have always had medical rationing and indeed, managed care organizations are imposing rationing on their subscribers, we must still address how we can do it fairly. How does alternative medicine look in this setting?

It is an ethical obligation of the health profession and society to employ available resources fairly. Physicians must act in the capacity of stewards in order to maximize benefits to patients and protect the limited resources of society. Thus, we must ask whether the treatments that go under the name alternative medicine represent the best use of resources. Are they the most economical and effective way to accomplish the goals of medicine? I submit if these treatments cannot withstand the test of empirical research, if their effectiveness could just as easily be explained by the "natural history of disease, regression to the mean, suggestion, counterirritation, distraction, expectation, consensus, the Stockholm effect (identifying with and aiding the desires of a dominant figure), fatigue, habituation, ritual, reinforcement, and other well-known psychological mechanisms,"[66] then we have wasted a lot of time and effort.

The time has been wasted on all the people who have spent years learning falsehoods about acupuncture points and the principles of homeopathy. And the patients have wasted their time, money and efforts receiving treatments that were not what they were represented to be or harmful. A counter-argument, of course, is that these elaborate rituals and symbols of healing are simply ways to "harness" the placebo effect in accordance with "expectancy theory," which has drawn the attention of both the scientific and popular press.[67,68,69] But are they the most efficient and effective ways—even this hypothesis can be and should be explored.

Otherwise how can we make rationing judgments in the absence of good data? As with all of medicine, we should test these practices by the same measure as we test medicine itself.

DEALING WITH PATIENTS

In the cases presented briefly at the beginning of this article we see examples of the potential conflict that sometimes occurs between the physician's professional integrity and the desire to honor the patient's personal values. How should the physician weigh this conflict?

I suggest the following steps:

First, just as any physician is obligated to seek information on all the factors that might reasonably affect a patient's illness and treatment, the physician should include as part of every patient's history an inquiry into the use of unconventional treatments—particularly now that we know how pervasive they are. The physician can easily and nonjudgmentally insert such questions into the routine inquiry about the patient's life activities, such as smoking, alcohol and caffeine intake, exercise, sexual activity, use of unprescribed drugs and vitamins, and so forth. This will be of increasing importance as it is likely within the next few decades more than half the people living in the United States will be of nonwhite ethnic background. For many of these patients unconventional therapies will have been handed down over many generations as part of religious or cultural practices or as traditions that arose out of coping with economic privation and lack of access to conventional medical care. Therefore, in gathering this information, it is particularly important to be sensitive and respectful. Success, of course, may depend in large part on how well the primary physician's institution itself has reached out and gained the trust of its various ethnic, social and religious communities.

Second, if the physician learns the patient is taking an unconventional treatment, such as a toxic herb[70,71] that presents a serious hazard to the patient's health, then the physician should not hesitate to recommend strongly against the treatment. Respect for multiculturalism should not be used as a sentimental excuse to abandon one's professional obligation to serve the patient's best interests. The physician's range of effort can extend from merely providing information (if that suffices) to negotiating and persuading (if that is successful) to seeking legal action (if that is warranted).

Third, if the patient is involved with an unconventional treatment that has a good chance of being beneficial, the physician should not disparage it simply because it is being provided by practitioners outside the AMA mainstream, for example chiropractors or massage therapists. One does not have to accept chiropractic theory that vertebral subluxation is the fundamental cause of disease[72] to acknowledge that spinal manipulation has been shown to be efficacious for acute low back pain[73,74,75]—although perhaps only marginally better than a less expensive educational intervention.[76] And massage therapy, unencumbered by Rolfing mumbo jumbo, has been adopted as part of standard treatments to alleviate musculoskeletal pain by a wide range of healthcare professionals because it is soothing, safe and noninvasive.

Fourth, if the unconventional treatment is neither useful or harmful, then the physician can exercise judgment in terms of the patient's best interests, keeping in mind both the patient's right to be informed and the potential benefit of the placebo effect. If the treatment is costly, for example if it involves a multitude of elaborate sessions, and is disproportionate to the patient's illness, the physician probably should express reservations, along with guiding the patient toward reliable information. Among the best currently available sources for gaining accurate information about alternative medical practices are the website www.quackwatch.com, and publications like the *Scientific Review of Alternative Medicine* and *Alternative Medicine Alert*.

By contrast, a recent review article published in a reputable medical journal lists selfserving alternative medicine organizations as "information resources" without providing more reliable, independent information sources.[77] The American Cancer Society[78] can be counted on for reliable evaluations of unconventional cancer treatments and The Arthritis Foundation[79] is a reliable source for information on quack arthritis treatments; however, the overall field of medicine is less well covered.

On the other hand, if the condition is serious and the treatment of negligible harm and cost, for example if the patient has terminal cancer and believes in green tea, the physician can easily agree to add whatever benefit this placebo effect offers to all the other components of good end-of-life care, which might include (in addition to skillful pain-management) prayer, imaging, meditation, music, art, and any number of other alternatives to medicine.

In all these instances, it is important the physician not reject or abandon the patient. Whatever the patient chooses to do is part of that patient's individuality and should be respected as such. A good physician would not refuse to care for a patient with heart disease or pulmonary disease just because the patient smoked, or abandon a diabetic patient who took too much pleasure in rich desserts.

And now to return to the specific cases. Both patients lack independent autonomy, hence decision-making capacity. I submit in the first case, the physician's duty to the patient is so strong that, failing to engage the parents' participation, the physician ought to be willing to employ legal measures to assure the patient, a minor, receives the necessary life-saving treatment. In the second case, since the present state of Alzheimer's drug treatment is, at best, marginally effective, I believe the physician can justifiably grant the family considerable leeway in allowing the unconventional treatments to be superimposed on and even substituted for conventional treatments if they do not adversely affect the patient's quality of life.

The most obvious difference, of course, is in the first case a life is threatened without appropriate treatment. One can sympathize with the parents' distress, but society (as represented by the court and child protective services) would almost certainly agree the parents are calculating risks and benefits in a way that threatens to subject their daughter to irrational neglect. Thus, when unconventional treatments lead to life-threatening consequences by diverting a patient from conventional treatments, the physician has good reason to call upon the notion of professional integrity, even if it means overriding the family's objections.

In the second case, the physician might consider making selective modifications to the duty of beneficence, which ordinarily mandates offering only those treatments that are considered efficacious. Although present-day drugs for Alzheimer's disease offer only modest benefits along with occasional toxicities, the primary physician knows that FDA-approved drugs have, at least, gone through preliminary safety and efficacy trials. By contrast, no such information has been gathered on the many unconventional treatments the family is accepting on behalf of the patient. Therefore, the physician might gain the family's confidence by agreeing to certain treatments, such as safe and pleasant non-toxic herbs and aromatherapy, meanwhile pointing out the lack of evidence, as well as unlikely placebo benefit (except perhaps on the family, which should not be discounted) associated with other treatments, such as therapeutic touch and Ayurveda.

It is important to remember that medicine is supposed to be a moral profession and, therefore, the principles that I have described should withstand popular and economic pressures. It distresses me when health-care leaders, policymakers, politicians—and alas, even physicians—use as their guiding principle not the search for good empirical data but rather "what the people want"[80] or what people (or insurance companies) are willing to pay. And although the contemporary Western medicine estab-lishment is often accused of exploiting its power, it is quite striking to me how much power the alternative medicine establishment has wielded throughout the country with so little demonstration of efficacy.

This is not to deny that alternative medicine is fulfilling important emotional needs of patients. And here we come to the observation I made earlier that we must seek reasons other than efficacy against disease to account for its popularity.

Twenty years ago, a UCSD medical student, Robert Avila, and I sur-veyed 100 persons in the San Francisco Bay area who were consulting homeopathic practitioners and asked them why.[81] These were not unso-phisticated people who were unaware of modem medicine. On the con-trary, we found them to be highly educated patients who were afflicted with difficult diseases—diseases that did not cure easily, such as chronic asthma and chronic arthritis. Their perceived needs, however, lay beyond the technology of medicine (which did not give them the cure they were hoping for).

Our survey taught us something important. Again and again, the patients emphasized that homeopathic practitioners would spend a great deal of time with them, going over their symptoms in meticulous detail before prescribing their treatment, all the while reinforcing that each person was a singular individual. This is in contrast to contemporary Western medicine which seeks to classify (and therefore lump) individuals within diagnostic categories. It became apparent to us these people, who were suffering from incurable illnesses (that remained uncured), were nevertheless made to feel better by practitioners who paid them such intense individual attention. Important emotional needs were being fulfilled—deeply human needs—by their homeopathic practitioners that were being neglected by science-based medicine. Were these practitioners (who probably would not acknowledge it) merely "harnessing" the placebo effect?

One could also argue for these patients (who probably would not acknowledge it either) the homeopathic practitioners were behaving very much like practitioners of a contemporary Western medical specialty, psychiatry, which is dedicated to addressing emotional needs and which admittedly has tolerated unsubstantiated theories and dubious healers. Indeed, managedcare organizations have been particularly intent on calling this specialty accountable in terms of outcome measures. Psychiatrists, in particular, are being penalized for spending far too much time with their patients. ("Is all that time and attention *really* necessary?") This scrutiny is all the more ironic since contemporary Western medical practice, which can now lay claim to demonstrable efficacy in the treatment of many severe emotional disorders, finds itself facing restrictions by the same managedcare organizations that are opening their arms to alternative medical practices that have demonstrated no such efficacy.

Finally, one human need we must also acknowledge is that throughout history human beings have been drawn toward magic and mysticism—and desperate patients toward snake oil and quackery. It is an inescapable part of the human condition. Again, it is particularly ironic in the modern era when science has replaced religion as a source of (arduously gained) "miracles," New Age healers—while roundly denouncing medicine—seek medicine's cover to make their own miraculous claims respectable. It is not alternative religion these practitioners are advertising but alternative medicine. Today, as noted above, many false messiahs come with M.D. degrees.

This point is worth emphasizing. There can be no doubt that religious belief provides spiritual comfort to many people, allowing them to connect personally through prayer to a transcendently experienced Supreme Being, while at the same time offering a pattern and purpose to life's mysteries, pains and sorrows. The right to have one's religious belief respected is therefore indisputable. The problem occurs when a personal belief becomes a generalized claim, either a forceful claimexpressed in bloody violence—that one's belief is The One True Faith; or when the belief is asserted as revealed truth exempt from skeptical inquiry, e.g., prayer cures cancer, AIDS is a result of "generations of sexual repression." It is in the latter area that I believe alternative medicine trespasses. Yes, alternative medical practitioners seem to fulfill deep human needs, but if they do so through unsubstantiated theories and dubious treatments they risk causing great harms to trusting patients.

Therefore, those of us who practice in the tradition of contemporary Western medicine must ask ourselves: What is our ethical responsibility? Are we contributing to those harms? As we move into the depersonalizing, timepressured, efficiency-oriented, corporate managedcare era, are we being so neglectful of our patients' needs, that *as a result of our neglect* we are *causing* our trusting patients to be lured toward those unsubstantiated theories and dubious treatments? This is the ethical problem that all of us practicing medicine today should take seriously.

NOTES

1. *Alternative Medicine: Expanding Medical Horizons (A Report to the National Institutes of Health on Alternative Medical Systems and Practices in the United States (Chantilly Report)*. Sept 14–16, 1992. Available through the Superintendent of Documents, P.O. Box 371954, Pittsburgh PA 15250-7954.

2. Bannerman RH. *Traditional Medicine and Healthcare Coverage*. World Health Organization, Geneva, 1983.

3. Brody JE. Alternative medicine makes inroads, but watch out for curves. *New York Times* 4/28/98, B10.

4. Eisenberg DM, Kessler RC, Foster C, et al. Unconventional medicine in the United States. Prevalence, costs, and patterns of use. *New England Journal of Medicine* 1993;328: 246–521.

5. See note 3, Brody 4/28/98, B10.

6. Elder NC, Gillcrist A, Minz R. Use of alternative health care by family practice patients. *Archives of Family Medicine* 1997;6:181-4.

7. Wetzel MS, Eisenberg DM, Kaptchuk Tj. Courses involving complementary and alternative medicine at US medical schools. *Journal of the American Medical Association* 1998;280:784-7.

8. Colgate MA. Gaining insurance coverage for alternative therapies. *Journal of Health Care Marketing* 1995;15:24,27.

9. Weber D. The mainstrearning of alternative medicine. *Healthcare Forum Journal* 1996;39(6):16-27.

10. Lagnado L. Oxford to create alternative-medicine network. *Wall Street Journal* 7 October 1996:A11.

11. Root-Bernstein R, Root-Bernstein M. *Honey, Mud, Maggots, and Other Medical Marvels.* New York: Houghton Mifflin Company, 1997; p. 255.

12. Wash. Rev. Code 48.43.045 (1996).

13. Deborah Senn, Insurance Commissioner, Every Category of Provider, Washington Office of Insurance Commissioner Bull. No. 95-9 (December 19, 1995).

14. Berthold HK, Sudhop T, Bertmann K. Effect of a garlic oil preparation on serum lipoproteins and cholesterol metabolism: A randomized controlled trial. *Journal of the American Medical Association* 1998;279:1900-02.

15. Curtius M. Touting garlic's glories. Despite study, Gilroy's devotion to aromatic crop is unshaken. *Los Angeles Times* 6/21/98, A3.

16. Fisher RA. *The Design of Experiments*, 7th ed. New York: Hafner, 1960.

17. Linde K, Clausius N, Ramirez G, et al. Are the clinical effects of home-opathy placebo effects? A meta-analysis of placebo-controlled trials. *Lancet* 1997;350:834-43.

18. Beyerstein BL, Downie S. Naturopathy. *The Scientific Review of Alternative Medicine* 1998;2(1):20-8.

19. Vickers AJ . Can acupuncture have specific effects on health? A systematic review of acupuncture antiemesis trials. *Journal of the Royal Society of Medicine* 1996;89:303 11.

20. ter Riet G, Kleiznen J, Knipschild P. Acupuncture and chronic pain: A criteria based meta-analysis. *Journal of Clinical Epidemiology* 1990;43:1191-99.

21. Rosa L, Rosa E, Sarner L. A close look at therapeutic touch. *Journal of the American Medical Association* 1998;279:1005-10.

22. 42 U.S.C. & 283g(b).

23. Acupuncture. NIH Consensus Statement 1997 November 3-5;15(5); in press. Available on the internet: http://odp.od.nih.gov/consensus/statements/cdc/107/107_stmt.html.

24. Cervantes FD, Schneiderman Lj. Anticoagulants in cerebrovascular disease: A critical review of studies. *Archives of Internal Medicine* 1975;135:875-7.

25. Eddy DM. Investigational treatments: How strict should we be? *Journal of the American Medical Association* 1997;278:179-85.

26. Dundee JS, Ghaly RG, Bill KM, et al. Effect of stimulation of the P6 antiemetic point on postoperative nausea and vomiting. *British Journal of Anaesthesia* 1989;63:612-8.

27. Dundee JW, McMillan C. Positive evidence for P6 acupuncture antiemesis. *Postgraduate Medicine Journal* 1991;67:417-22.

28. Eisenberg DM. Advising patients who seek alternative medical therapies. *Annals of Internal Medicine* 1997;127:61-69.

29. See note 19, Vickers 1996;89:303-11.

30. See note 20, ter Riet G, Kleiznen J, Knipschild P 1990:43:1191-99.

31. Colditz GA, Miller JN, Mosteller F. How study design affects outcomes in comparisons of therapy. *Statistics in Medicine* 1989;8:441-54.

32. Schulz KF, Chalmers I, Hayes R.J. Empirical evidence of bias: Dimensions of methodological quality associated with estimates of treatment effects in controlled trials. *Journal of the American Medical Association* 1995;273:408 12.

33. Khan K, Daya S, Jadad A. The importance of quality of primary studies in producing unbiased systematic reviews. *Archives of Internal Medicine* 1996;156:661-6.

34. See note 20, ter Riet G, Kleiznen J, Knipschild P 1990:43:1191-99.

35. Gifford RH, Feinstein AR. A critique of methodology in studies of anticoagulant therapy for acute myocardial infarction. *New England Journal of Medicine* 1969:280:351-7.

36. See Note 25, Eddy 1997;278:179-85.

37. Portions of the following section were previously published in slightly different form in: Schneiderman J. Medical ethics and alternative medicine. *The Scientific Review of Alternative Medicine* 1998;2(1):63-6.

38. Beauchamp TL, Childress JF. *Principles of Biomedical Ethics*, 2nd ed. New York: Oxford University Press, 1983.

39. Ellis J, Mulligan 1, Rowe J, Sackett DL. Inpatient general medicine is evidence based. *Lancet* 1995;346:407-10.

40. Institute of Medicine. *Assessing Medical Technologies*. National Academy Press. Washington, D.C. 1985.

41. Gill P, Dowell AC, Neal RD, Smith N, Heywood P, Wilson AE. Evidence based general practice: A retrospective study of interventions in one training practice. *British Medical Journal* 1996;312:819-21.

42. Michaud G ' McGowan JL, van der Jagt R, Wells G, Tugwell P. Are therapeutic decisions supported by evidence from health care research? *Archives of Internal Medicine* 1998;158:1665-8.

43. Chopra D. *Quantum Healing*. New York: Bantam Books, 1989. p. 240.

44. Northrup C. *Women's Bodies, Women's Wisdom*. New York: Bantam Books, 1995.

45. Weil A. *Spontaneous Healing*. New York: Fawcett Columbine, 1995; 235-7.

46. Hilts PJ. Severe Side Effects Are Seen in Experimental AIDS Drug. *New York Times* September 27, 1989, A15.

47. Moser HW. Suspended judgment: Reactions to the motion picture "Lorenzo's Oil." *Controlled Clinical Trials* 1994;15:161-4.

48. Zinkham WH, Kickler T, Borel J. Lorenzo's oil and thrombocytopenia in patients with adrenoleukodystrophy. *New England Journal of Medicine* 1993;328:1124-5.

49. Schneiderman LJ, Jecker NS. Is the treatment beneficial, experimental or futile? *Cambridge Quarterly of Healthcare Ethics* 1996;5:248-256.

50. Altman LK. Drug mixture curbs HIV in lab, doctors report, but urge caution. *New York Times*, Feb. 18, 1993, A1.

51. Lannin DR, Matthews HF, Mitchell J. Influence of socioeconomic and cultural factors on racial differences in late-stage presentation of breast cancer. *Journal of the American Medical Association* 1998;279:1801-7.

52. Mitchell JM, Scott E. Physician ownership of physical therapy services: Effects on charges, utilization, profits, and service characteristics. *Journal of the American Medical Assocation* 1992;268:2055-59.

53. Mitchell JM, Sunshine JH. Consequences of physicians' ownership of health care facilities—joint ventures in radiation therapy. *New England Journal of Medicine* 1992;327:1497-501.

54. Swedlow A, Johnson G, Mithline N, et al. Increased costs and rates of use in the California workers' compensation system as a result of self-referral by physicians. *New England Journal of Medicine* 1992;327:1502-6.

55. Council on Ethical and judicial Affairs, American Medical Association. Conflicts of interest: Physician ownership of medical facilities. *Journal of the American Medical Association* 1992;67:2366-9.

56. Council on Ethical and judicial Affairs, American Medical Association. Conflicts of interest: Physician ownership of medical facilities. *Journal of the American Medical Association* 1992;67:2366-9.

57. Dundee JS, Ghaly RG, Bill KM, et al. Effect of stimulation of the P6 antiemetic point on postoperative nausea and vomiting. *British Journal of Anaesthesia* 1989;63:612-8.

58. Dundee JW, McMillan C. Positive evidence for P6 acupuncture antiemesis. *Postgraduate Medicine Journal* 1991;67:417-22.

59. Moore ME, Berk SN. Acupuncture for chronic shoulder pain: an experimental study with attention to the role of placebo and hypnotic susceptibility. *Annals of Internal Medicine* 1976;84:381-384.

60. Helms JM. An overview of medical acupuncture. *Alternative Therapies in Health and Medicine* 1998;4:35-45.

61. Gravitz MA. Early uses of hypnosis as surgical anesthesia. *American Journal of Clinical Hypnosis* 1988;30:201-8.

62. Angell M, Kassirer JP. Alternative medicine—the risks of untested and unregulated remedies. *New England Journal of Medicine* 1998;339:839-41.

63. Canedy D. Real medicine or medicine show? Growth of herbal remedy sales raises issues about value. *New York Times* July 23, 1998; C1, C4.

64. See note 63, Canedy July 23, 1998; C1, C4.

65. See note 63, Canedy July 23,1998; C1, C4.

66. Sampson W. On the National Institute of Drug Abuse Consensus Conference on acupuncture. *The Scientific Review of Alternative Medicine* 1998;2(l):54-5.

67. Blakeslee S. Placebos prove so powerful even experts are surprised. *New York Times* October 13, 1998; F1, F4.

68. Brown WA. The placebo effect. Scientific American January 1998;90-5.

69. Saintonge M C de, Herxheimer A. Harnessing placebo effects in health care. *Lancet* 1994;344(8928):995-8.

70. Newall CA, Anderson LA, Phillipson JD. *Herbal Medicines: A Guide for Health Care Professionals*. London: Pharmaceutical Press, 1996.

71. Wilkinson JA. The internet as a research and information tool for herbal medicine. *British Journal of Phytotherapy* 1995;4:34-45.

72. Crelin ES. Chiropractic. In Stalker D, Glymour C (eds.) *Examining-Holistic Medicine*. Amherst, N.Y.: Prometheus Books, 1989.

73. Bigos SJ, Bowyer O, Braea G, et al. Acute low back pain problems in adults: Clinical Practice Guideline No. 14, Rockville, MD; U.S. Department of Health and Human Services, Public Health Service, Agency for Health Care Policy and Research, AHCPR publication No. 95-0642,1992.

74. Shekelle PG, Adams AH, Chassin MR, Hurwitz EL, Brook RH. Spinal manipulation for low-back pain. *Annals of Internal Medicine* 1992;117:590-8.

75. Shekelle PG, Coulter I, Hurwitz EL, et al. Congruence between decisions to initiate chiropractic spinal manipulation for low back pain and appropriateness criteria in North Ameica. *Annals of Internal Medicine* 1998;129:9-17.

76. Cherkin DC, Deyo RA, Battie M, Street J, Barlow W. A comparison of physical therapy, chiropractice manipulation, and provision of an educational booklet for the treatment of patients with low back pain. *New England Journal of Medicine* 1998;339:1021-9.

77. See note 28, Eisenberg 1997;127:61-9.

78. http://www.cancer.org/frames.html.

79. The Arthritis Foundation. Atlanta, GA. (404) 872-7100. Ask for the information line.

80. Schneiderman LJ. Commentary: Bringing clarity to the futility debate: Are the cases wrong? *Cambridge Quarterly of Healthcare Ethics* 1998;7(3):273-8.

81. Avina RL, Schneiderman LJ. Why patients choose homeopathy. *Western Journal of Medicine* 1978;128:366-9.

14

THERAPEUTIC TOUCH
What Could Be the Harm?

Dónal P. O'Mathúna

THERAPEUTIC TOUCH (TT) IS AN ALTERNATIVE THERAPY ORIGINALLY developed in the early 1970s by Dora Kunz and Dolores Krieger, R.N., Ph.D. Kunz, a self-declared clairvoyant, was then president of the Theosophical Society in America. This quasireligious group mixes Eastern religions, mysticism, and the occult and remains an active promoter of TT through its publisher, Quest Publications, and its annual conference held at Pumpkin Hollow Farm. Krieger was on the faculty at New York University's School of Nursing and did much to popularize TT among nurses through teaching and writing.

In the United States and Canada, TT is taught at 75 schools and universities, and practiced at 95 health facilities.[1] Krieger claims she has personally taught the technique to more than 48,000 healthcare professionals in 75 countries.[2] Nursing organizations like the Nurse Healers-Professional Associates, Inc., actively promote TT's use in clinical settings. The American Nurses Association, American Holistic Nurses Association, and the National League for Nursing promote TT to various extents through accredited workshops and publications. The North American Nursing Diagnosis Association has accepted the nursing diagnosis "energy-field disturbance," for which TT is the only treatment recommended.[3] Not only has the Office of Complementary and Alternative Medicine funded TT research, but the U.S. Department of Defense gave a $355,000 grant to nursing researchers at the University of Alabama to study TT.[4]

Alternative therapies are generally promoted as less harmful because they are more natural and gentle. However, this is not necessarily the case, as the harmful effects of herbal remedies clearly demonstrate. Yet because of the association of natural and harmless, investigation into potential harmful effects of alternative therapies has been neglected.[5] This article will demonstrate that there is sufficient reason from the literature of TT practitioners to be concerned about TT's harmful effects. Healthcare providers should be aware of these because of their ethical implications in the promotion, teaching, and practice of TT.

THE BASICS OF TT

Some understanding of TT itself is necessary before examining its potentially harmful effects. Most would agree that someone's touch can be comforting and beneficial, especially when ill or anxious. However, TT does not involve physical touch. According to Krieger, it involves "the conscious use of the hands to direct or modulate, for therapeutic purposes, selected nonphysical human energies that activate the physical body."[6] This life energy is the same as Hindu *prana*, Chinese *qi* or *chi*, and ancient Egyptian *ka*.[7] Thus, TT is another alternative therapy based on vitalistic notions of human life energy, referred to as "life energy" in this article.

Krieger acknowledged in 1979 that while TT involved the assessment and transfer of life energy, "It should be said quite frankly that there is little support that this actually occurs, for at this time there are no accepted means of measuring this transfer. . . . The same must be said about the modulating of energy. . . ."[8] Nothing had changed by 1994 when Janet Quinn, R.N., Ph.D., a prominent TT promoter, was reported as stating that "we don't have empirical data to demonstrate the existence of a personal energy field. It's a working hypothesis."[9]

The practice of TT generally moves through five phases. First, practitioners enter a state of meditation, called centering. "Centering is an act of self-searching, a going within to explore the deeper levels of yourself. . . . In centering, you relate to the extraordinary stillness of the personal, private world within you, and you bask in its profoundly quieting psychological and physical effects."[10] When centered, practitioners have a "decisive shift in consciousness"[11] which allows them to detect life energy. Practitioners must remain centered throughout TT to gain understanding of their own and others' life energy, "reflected from the deep places of your inner self."[12]

Once properly centered, practitioners begin the second phase, called assessment. The patient sits or lies comfortably while practitioners pass their hands over the patient's body without making contact. Although some practitioners include physical touch, the literature maintains that hands should be kept a few inches above the skin. It is believed that highly sensitive "chakras" extend from everyone's hands. These non-physical "transformers" convert human energy into the physically detectable forms of energy and matter of people's bodies.[13]

During assessment, information about the patient's life energy is gathered. Another assumption is that life energy forms a "human energy field." When this is balanced and symmetrical, the person is healthy; when unbalanced, illness results. Imbalances are detected during the assessment phase as a variety of "cues," such as "vague hunches, passing impressions, flights of fancy, or, in precious moments, true insights or intuitions."[14] During this phase, "a good reason or a strong, irresistible, intuitive urge"[15] is experienced to determine which form of treatment is given during the third and fourth phases.

After assessment, imbalances in the energy field are corrected. During the third phase, called "unruffling," practitioners sweep their hands over the length of the patient's body in long, rhythmic strokes. These smooth out the energy field and remove areas of "congestion." Simultaneously, the patient is instructed in visualization to help develop healing imagery. Unruffling is also said to clear "energy blockages" which prepares the energy field for the treatment phase.

Treatment occurs in the fourth phase when practitioners send energy to the patient to correct specific imbalances detected earlier. Various techniques are used here, all guided by what is called "the simple principle of opposites."[16] Whatever type of "cue" is detected during assessment, its opposite is sent during treatment. For example, if an area of hotness is sensed in the energy field, practitioners visualize coolness while sending energy to that area. If irregular rhythms are detected in the flow of energy, a synchronous form of energy would be projected during treatment. Practitioners visualize projecting the energy through their hand chakras by " 'effortless effort' that is guided by conscious, mindful action."[17] Practitioners must also remain properly centered and focused completely on intending to help and heal. The fifth and final phase is reached when practitioners determine it is time to stop. At this point, the patient's energy field is reassessed to evaluate the degree to which the energy field has been balanced.

According to Krieger, TT's most reliable clinical effect is causing a relaxation response in the patient within two to four minutes. The second most reliable clinical effect "is the amelioration or eradication of pain. . . . For Therapeutic Touch's third most reliable clinical effect, I would choose the facilitation of the healing process per se."[18] As an example of the latter, she claimed (without citation) that several replicated studies found that bone fractures heal more than twice as quickly when treated with TT

Krieger also presented anecdotal reports of TT relieving many conditions, including premenstrual syndrome, depression, complications in premature babies, and secondary infections due to HIV.[19] Another practitioner claimed that, "Therapeutic Touch consistently demonstrated an ability to lower blood pressure, decrease edema, ease abdominal cramps and nausea, resolve fevers, stimulate growth in premature infants and accelerate the healing process in fractures and in some wounds and other infections."[20] Most dramatically, Krieger claimed that in "several cases" premature babies who "in spite of heroic medical measures . . . had been extubated and declared dead" were resuscitated when given TT and went on to complete recoveries.[21]

Such impressive claims arc often difficult to accept in light of the standard medical model and the different assumptions and procedures involved in TT. Yet, as was stated earlier, TT has become very popular across the nursing profession, and is starting to receive interest from some physicians.[22] With such growing popularity it is imperative that studies on the efficacy and safety of TT be reported accurately. Research on TT's efficacy has been conducted for over twenty-five years, but the results are often not supportive of the claims made for it.[23,24] Those studies with positive results are often methodologically flawed, or later fail replication. Yet in spite of this, proponents continue to claim that TT is research-supported.

HARM TO PATIENTS

This article will focus on concerns that TT might cause various harms. Many TT practitioners claim it does not cause harm. Some claim it cannot cause harm. It is difficult to see how moving one's hands a few inches above a patient's body could cause physical harm. Krieger admitted that, "The idea that pain can be created with Therapeutic Touch may be surprising."[25] However, she went on to describe an exercise whereby practitioners could demonstrate the painful effects by treating one another while disregarding the receiver's tolerance level. It seems that those who accept the therapeutic benefits of TT should be easily able to appreciate its harmful effects.

As early as 1979 Krieger cautioned that energy should be sent carefully to the patient during the treatment phase. "It is not enough to channel energy to an ill person; as a matter of experience, it seems that one can actually do more harm than good by simply flooding a weakened person with energy.[26] She stressed the importance of practicing TT according to her guidelines so that its safety record would be maintained. By 1993, Krieger was more specific: "Human energies are not well understood at this time, but we do know that indiscriminate and persistent interaction can overload the human system; a healee can overdose on human energies."[27] She described some of the symptoms: "The progressive signs of overload to be aware of include increasing restlessness, irritability, and anxiety that may be expressed as hostility or felt as pain by the healee."[28] She noted that two people doing TT simultaneously on one patient must exercise caution. "Otherwise, the healee may experience ill effects such as nausea, dizziness, or irritability."[29]

Other general warnings have been given.[30] Another proponent was more specific: "By performing a long heating touch session on someone with a cold, you can trigger an even deeper discharge or elimination of waste products, and thus intensify the symptoms and cause more suffering. . . . In other words, you will increase the suffering of the patient significantly."[31] She then warned that when patients have a fever or inflammation: "Do not send life force into the body initially. This will serve to further inflame the condition."[32] And again: "When treating people with cancer, *do not send energy to the area of the tumor*. This will only serve to strengthen the disease and make it more virulent"[33] (emphasis original).

While no studies were given to support these cautions, they demonstrate the serious concerns that some proponents have about TT's potential harm. However, two studies found statistical significance for slower wound-healing rates after patients received TT (contradicting earlier studies). The researcher hypothesized: "Prior anecdotal research has indicated that if the healer is emotionally upset or physically ill, a transference of the state from practitioner to the patient might occur, thereby resulting in not only a nonsignificant treatment effect but, in extreme cases, a disturbance or inhibition of the patient's normal rate of healing."[34] If patients are told they will be receiving life energy, they should also be told of the possibility of getting "negative energy."

Leading proponents also note that certain groups of patients are more sensitive to TT than others. In 1979, Krieger reiterated Dora Kunzs warning that TT ought be done very gently and for no more than two to three minutes on children, very old people, very debilitated people, and in treating any person's head.[35] Another author claimed, "However, children's systems are very sensitive, and as with medication, therapeutic touch must be given in smaller, more gentle doses. Too much or incorrect repatterning can cause discomfort, so it is extremely important to be sensitive to the patient's responses."[36] Concerns for these same groups of patients were reiterated more recently.[37] Again, no studies have been cited to support these concerns, although one study found increased anxiety among elderly hospitalized patients given TT compared to a control group, and cautioned against using TT with the elderly.[38]

All these cautions indicate that research into potential harmful effects of TT is needed. Until rigorous studies show that these concerns are unwarranted, TT providers should inform trainees, patients, and research subjects about these harmful effects. Yet precisely the opposite occurs. For example, Krieger specifically cautioned those using TT with burn victims: "Burns are very sensitive to energy overload, so Therapeutic

Touch must be done very gently at the site of burned tissue. Do the work for very short periods—two to three minutes at a time—and keep your hands moving so that your hand chakras do not focus energy too intensely at the burn site."[39]

The U.S. Department of Defense funded a study on the use of TT with burn victims. No mention of these potentially harmful effects was made in the grant proposal, although Krieger's book with the warnings was cited elsewhere. Treatment lengths from five to twenty minutes were proposed, with no mention of Krieger's concerns. The informed consent given to research subjects stated: "There is no risk of injury from the administrations of TT."[40] Other informed consents are similar. One from a research project involving children stated: "In no case have there ever been any negative effects associated with TT. . . . There are no known risks."[41] Another from a project with the elderly stated: "Therapeutic touch has no known negative side effects."[42] These statements contradict TT's own literature.

Even if TT works as a placebo, it could still cause harm. Contrary to the view that placebos are harmless sugar pills, they can cause problems known as "nocebo effects." These sometimes exacerbate preexisting symptoms or produce pain in healthy subjects. One review of 109 studies found adverse effects in 19 percent of patients given placebos. "Headaches were reported by 70 percent of students told that a (nonexistent) electric current was passing through their heads.[43] If nonexistent electric currents cause headaches, what might (nonexistent?) life energy cause? Regardless, the power of suggestion and psychological effects deserve more respect than is granted by a flippant "It can't do any harm."

If research projects are undertaken and funded based on the experiences of TT experts, then those same people's concerns about the harmful effects need to be taken seriously. Medical ethics places a high value on informed consent. Research subjects must be told about potential harm before deciding to participate in a research project. Patients should also be told of these harms and the fact that they have not yet been adequately researched. Only then can patients' rights to make informed decisions be upheld.

HARM TO PRACTITIONERS

In addition to harmful effects on patients, statements have been made that practitioners may experience negative effects. These are explained on the basis of a two-way flow of energy. "It is also important for you to remain centered and aware of your own reactions to the healing process to not absorb any unbalanced energy from your patient."[44] Another proponent stated: "If you're not centered, you may actually absorb the patient's negative energy. That's why novices to this modality sometimes report post-treatment headaches."[45]

"Centering" is a form of meditation.[46] It could therefore produce the side-effects of meditation. One study found that 48 percent of Transcendental Meditation (TM) practitioners reported adverse effects from meditation.[47] The most common negative effects reported were anxiety, depression, confusion, frustration, mental and physical tension, and inexplicable outbursts of antisocial behavior. These were reported by TM trainers who persisted with the method, not people who had stopped practicing. Other studies report similar findings, with documented cases of adverse effects as serious as attempted suicide and psychiatric hospitalization.[48] All these occurred from "simply" practicing meditation.

TT practitioners are encouraged to include visualization in their meditation and practice. According to a proponent of these practices: "At the initial state of meditation, a cultivator often experiences emotional instability, physical abnormalities, and hallucinations. . . . The Tendai Buddhist meditation tradition, *shikan*, calls this the state of '*majikyo*' (the demonic realm). . . . The Zen-sickness discussed by Zen Buddhism is probably also the same." Two other proponents cautioned: "All too often those who recommend various meditation and visualization practices have no or only limited experience with them, and may have no knowledge at all of their possible negative ramifications."[50] They elaborated: "Visualization is never innocuous. . . . What is important to realize in this connection is that ignorance does not always protect us from harm. . . . [M]editators who are inexperienced in discerning truth from fiction or actual reality from hallucination . . . may think they have contacted some pure realm of existence or some deity or spiritual master when, in fact, they have only encountered the clever productions of their own mind."[51]

Manipulation of life energy, or prana, is also a part of occult and magical healing practices. A proponent warned of "The dangers incident to working with the fires or with the pranas of the Universe."[52] A physician who promotes these practices also cautioned about involvement with life energy: "Tapping these energies is fire, and the consequences are serious and can be dangerous. . . . The consequences of immature judgment, of toying with the chakra system, can be psychosis, aggravation of neuroses, acceleration of disease processes and suicide."[53]

A past president of the Theosophical Society in America, prior to Kunz, claimed that magnetic healing, laying-on of hands, and absent healing were various ways to manipulate life energy, which he called magnetism. He cautioned against all these practices, which his society now promotes: "I think it is a very dangerous thing for a man, even with the best of motives, to attempt to use his magnetism upon another human being. I know that good can be done. But I also know that evil can be worked. I know there are noble-minded men who do heal; but I think it extremely dangerous. I would not allow it on me. . . . No man is wise enough to he able to touch the mind or even the body of another being magnetically. It is playing with fire. . . . Magnetic healing really is but another form of hypnotism or psychologization, call it what you like; and this can be, and often is, made a devil's work; so much so that there are laws today in most civilized countries against the indiscriminate practice of hypnotism, particularly in medical schools."[54]

These cautions are probably based in observations of factual events. They demonstrate the concern those intimately familiar with Eastern and occult traditions have about those who dabble in practices they don't fully understand. Problems from these techniques have led to the establishment of the Spiritual Emergence Network. This international organization has 1,100 trained counselors (many with Ph.D., M.D., or MSW degrees), operating out of 40 centers, to help people through what it describes as spiritual emergencies.[55] These can be precipitated by ordinary events like the death of a loved one or divorce, but also by what it calls transpersonal events. These occur when "people are brought into more direct and conscious relationship to their own life force, or prana in Sanskrit. It is not unusual to sense vibrations and streaming energy in the body, or even to see these manifestations of life energy in other people or natural elements."[56]

These metaphysical terms probably describe acute depressive episodes and hallucinatory events. They can produce disorientation, confusion, and isolation, leading to severe depression and anxiety states, with resulting hospitalization for psychiatric problems.[57] Various forms of energy healing have precipitated these events in either the practitioner, the patient, or both. Although studies have not shown that TT causes these effects, anecdotal reports of such problems exist and deserve further scrutiny.

Krieger wants TT to become a common event in every family. Before introducing people to TT and its form of meditation, the possible dangers and discomforts need to be investigated further. Those responsible for offering courses in TT should be aware of these dangers, inform students of them, and know how to respond to any psychiatric problems. Again, informed consent requires that these harms be discussed before people consent to participate in the practice.

HOLISTIC HARM

TT is part of the move to a more holistic approach to health and healing. The holistic approach views people as more than isolated, physical individuals. Yet ironically, these approaches often fail to address risks and harms from a holistic perspective, and often reveal a materialistic definition of harm. Concerns about physical harm are important, but the potential for psychological, intellectual, spiritual, and financial harm must also be examined. The broader "holistic harm" must be addressed.

A nursing editorial on TT addressed one aspect of this: "The harm, very simply, is that when we use nursing time and resources for such practices our clients may not receive the kind of sound care they want and need."[58] Wasting resources is both harmful and unjust, leaving fewer resources available in an already overextended system. Pressure exists throughout the current healthcare system to cut expenditures. Providing "low tech" alternative therapies may seem an attractive solution. A number of managedcare organizations already provide coverage for selected alternative therapies, and 58 percent of national health-maintenance organizations plan to do so by the end of 1998.[59]

Decisions about whether or not to provide any form of treatment should be based on the best evidence available for its effectiveness. This will diminish the harm of offering unsafe or ineffective treatments, or drawing patients away from effective treatments. Yet at a symposium on integrating alternative therapies into managedcare plans, proponents acknowledged there was little evidence for their effectiveness. They called for coverage of alternative therapies based on patient demand and the potential for profit. The physician-manager of one group's alternativemedicine division stated: "I believe that if the competitors don't listen to what their customers are saying and enter this [alternative medicine] market they are going to lose a lot of business, and I'm going to take it from them."[60]

A second indirect, but no less pervasive, harm that can occur from the promotion of TT is a devaluation of health care based on objective evidence and science.[61] As stated earlier, proponents admit no scientific evidence exists for human energy fields. Peer reviews of TT research have consistently found a lack of evidence for its efficacy. Yet TT proponents respond by claiming that critiques reveal more about the biases of science than TT's lack of efficacy.[62]

An article in a nursing journal claimed that alternative therapies are opposed by scientific paradigms which are "male dominated, exclusive, authoritarian, linear, and rigid."[63] These lead, according to another article, to "reductionist medicine" which results in "continued disease, dependence on 'management' with drugs and surgery (control over nature being a fundamental need of patriarchal science), poor quality of life, and tremendous cost to patient and community."[64] In other words, scientific medicine is the source of all modern health care's problems. Only by rejecting the scientific method and stressing experience and inner guidance can a more healing, caring form of health care be realized.

Rather than criticize TT an influential nursing textbook encouraged nurses to accept it as a way to "celebrate the diversity among us."[65] The search for research supporting TT's effectiveness is merely a social construct of Western culture. Noting that TT is rooted in Eastern philosophy, this textbook dismissed the need for research because: "The Eastern mind does not care how it works, only that it does."[66] Yet the crucial question of how anyone can know something works was not addressed. These advocates of postmodernism assert that science offers only one among many socially constructed views of reality; and each is equally valid. The claims of science, even about physical reality, are seen as no more reliable than those arising from intuition, personal experience, and feelings.[67]

What would be the consequences if healthcare decisions were based on these criteria? All drugs could be accepted since earlier drug testing was done by white, male, European scientists, and thus was socially biased. The only evidence needed to promote a new procedure would he someone claiming, "It worked for me." Since some procedures are used which have not been proved by blinded clinical trials, all procedures should be available for patients to choose.[68] Snake oil, bloodletting, and anesthesia using whiskey could be offered to patients as a way to assure openness to diversity.

Scientific medicine has made mistakes, ignored its limitations, and not been consistently applied. But it has also delivered dramatic benefits to the physical health of millions of people around the world. The world needs better application of scientific principles to all aspects of health care, as is occurring in the move toward evidence-based medicine. Much harm will occur if scientific principles are not valued and rigorously applied to healthcare issues.

The third form of "holistic harm" arises from TT's religious origins. Although said to be based on the biblical laying-on of hands, TT differs from it dramatically. Rather, TT has its origins in other religions. Krieger, a Buddhist, admits that TT is based on the same principles as Buddhism.[69] A practice identical to TT, but called auric or pranic healing, is found in Western occult and Wiccan religions.[70,71] This becomes problematic, if not harmful, when patients are exposed to TT without first being informed of its religious connections. Patients have been offended to discover this connection after being given TT.

The harm from TT's religious connections has been recognized by the Equal Employment Opportunity Commission. One policy states that employees cannot be required to learn or practice TT if they believe it conflicts with their religious beliefs.[72] Other "New Age" practices integral to TT, such as meditation, guided visualization, and inducing altered states of consciousness, are also specified in the policy. Commenting on this policy, a law professor stated: "New Age training programs have the potential to create an intimidating work environment. According to judicial interpretation, the term religious includes the new age philosophy and new age training programs. Although, new age consultants and employers argue such training programs are not religious, the courts will likely hold otherwise. Most new age training courses are derived from Eastern religions, such as Buddhism and Hinduism."[73]

While alternative practitioners promote spirituality as if it were morally neutral, most religious traditions claim there are true and false beliefs about the spiritual realm. Many also claim there are good and evil spiritual powers, with the latter capable of causing spiritual harm. Our postmodern culture claims that all beliefs are equally valid (or invalid, depending on one's overall perspective). Yet the recent tragedy of the Heaven's Gate Cult group demonstrates that beliefs have effects, and that actions based on some erroneous beliefs, can be harmful. If health is to he viewed holistically, to the extent that we base our lives on truth, we will be healthy.

If employers promoting TT have a legal duty to accommodate their employees' religious convictions, TT practitioners have an ethical duty to inform patients and research subjects of potential religious conflicts. This also raises interesting questions about the appropriateness of teaching TT at state institutions, or providing TT at government-run healthcare facilities, especially if it were established that government resources were being used to promote certain religious perspectives.

CONCLUSION

Contrary to the claims of proponents that TT is a harmless therapy, there are sufficient concerns in practitioners' own literature to warrant informing students and patients of the potential harms. While these concerns are anecdotal, they warrant rigorous investigation if TT continues to be practiced. The lack of physical contact in TT makes its ability to cause harm difficult to understand. However, research on adverse effects from meditation suggests that TT's harmful effects may originate in centering and the psychological states induced in patients.

The more subtle forms of "holistic harm" are no less problematic. Healthcare systems will always need to change and improve. But minimizing science and objective standards will cause further harm. Studies on TT may reveal that patients benefit from having caring people spend time with them focused on their well-being. Only rigorous scientific Studies will show whether the cause is the human interaction or some life-energy exchange. People need to be informed of the notions under-lying TT, its lack of efficacy, its potential for causing harm, and its religious nature. Given this information, they can decide whether or not to indulge in it. Harm arises when they are not given all the information needed to make an informed decision.

NOTES

1. Krieger D. *Therapeutic Touch Inner Workbook: Ventures in Transpersonal Healing*. Santa Fe, NM: Bear & Company; 1997.

2. Horrigan B. Dolores Krieger, RN, PhD: Healing with Therapeutic Touch. *Alt Ther*. 1998;4:87-92.

3. Carpentio LJ. *Nursing Diagnosis: Application to Clinical Practice*. 6th ed. Philadelphia, PA: Lippincott; 1995:355-358.

4. Turner JG. *The Effect of Therapeutic Touch on Pain and Infection in Burn Patients*. 1994. Tri-Service Nursing Research Grant #MDA 905-94-Z-0080 and Application #N94-020.

5. Ernst E. The ethics of complementary medicine. *J Med Ethics*. 1996;22:197-198.

6. Krieger D. *Accepting Your Power to Heal: The Personal Practice of Therapeutic Touch*. Santa Fe, NM: Bear & Company; 1993:3-4.

7. Ibid., p. 112.

8. Krieger D. The Therapeutic Touch: How to Use Your Hands to Help or to Heal. Englewood Cliffs, NJ: Prentice-Hall; 1979:57.

9. Jaroff L. A no-touch therapy. *Time*. November 21, 1994:89.

10. Krieger, *Accepting Your Power to Heal*, p. 17.

11. Krieger, *Therapeutic Touch Inner Workbook*, p. 21.

12. Krieger, *Accepting Your Power to Heal*, p. 18.

13. Krieger, *Therapeutic Touch Inner Workbook*, p. 5 1.

14. Krieger, *Accepting Your Power to Heal*.

15. Ibid., p. 29.

16. Ibid., p. 46.

17. Ibid., p. 12.

18. Ibid., pp. 83-84.

19. Ibid., pp. 133-172.

20. Thorpe B. Touch: a modality missing from your practice? *Adv Nurs Pract.* 1994;2: 10.

21. Krieger, *Therapeutic Touch Inner Workbook*, p. 12.

22. Goldman EL. New Age therapies are put to the test. *Intern Med News.* November 1, 199 5; 1,3 3.

23. Clark PE, Clark MJ. Therapeutic Touch: is there a scientific basis for the practice? *Nurs Res.* 1984;33:37-41.

24. Claman FIN. *Report of the Chancellor's Committee on Therapeutic Touch.* Denver, CO: University of Colorado Health Sciences Center; 1994.

25. Krieger, *Accepting Your Power to Heal*, p. 7 5,

26. Krieger, *The Therapeutic Touch*, p. 60.

27. Krieger, *Accepting Your Power to Heal*, p. 169.

28. Ibid., p. 75, cf. 74.

29. Ibid., p. 128.

30. Mackey R. Discover the healing power of Therapeutic Touch. *Am J Nurs.* April 1995;95:27-32.

31. Cowens D. *A Gift for Healing: How You Can Use Therapeutic Touch.* New York: Crown Trade Paperbacks; 1996:56-57.

32. Ibid., p. 208.

33. Ibid., p. 209.

34. Wirth DP. Complementary healing intervention and dermal wound reepithelialization: an overview. *Int Journal Psychosom.* 1995;42:5 1 .

35. Krieger, *The Therapeutic Touch*, p. 5 5.

36. Macrae J. Therapeutic Touch in practice. *Am J Nurs.* April 1979;79:665.

37. Wytias CA. Therapeutic Touch in primary care. *Nurs Pract Forum.* June 1994;5:91-97.

38. Parkes BS. *Therapeutic Touch as an Intervention to Reduce Anxiety in Elderly Hospitalized Patients.* Austin, TX: University of Texas at Austin;1985. Dissertation.

39. Krieger, *Accepting Your Power to Heal*, p. 75.

40. Turner JG. *The Effect of Therapeutic Touch on Pain and Infection.*

41. France NEM. *A Phenomenological Inquiry on the Child's Lived Experience of Perceiving the Human Energy Field using Therapeutic Touch.* Denver, CO: University of Colorado; 1991:211. Dissertation.

42. Parkes BS, *Therapeutic Touch as an Intervention*, pp. 95-96.

43. Turner JA, Deyo RA, Loeser JD, Von Korff M, Fordyce WE. The importance of placebo effects in pain treatment and research. *JAMA*. 1994;271:1609-1614.

44. Wytias, Therapeutic Touch in primary care, p. 94.

45. Mackey, Discover the healing power of Therapeutic Touch, p. 28.

46. Macrae J. Therapeutic Touch as meditation. In: *Spiritual Aspects of the Healing Arts*. Wheaton, IL: Theosophical Publishing House; 1985:272-288.

47. Otis LS. Adverse effects of Transcendental Meditation. In: Shapiro DH Jr., Walsh RN, eds. *Meditation: Classic and Contemporary Perspectives*. New York, NY: Aldone; 1984:201-207.

48. Shapiro DH Jr. Adverse effects of meditation: a preliminary investigation of long-term meditators. *Int J Psychosom*. 1992;29: 62-66.

49. Yasuo Y. *The Body: Toward an Eastern Mind-Body Theory*. Albany, NY: State University of New York Press; 1987:215.

50. Zangpo S, Feuerstein G. The risks of visualization: growing roots can be dangerous. *Quest*. Summer 1995;2630,84.

51. Ibid., pp. 28-29.

52. Bailey AA. *Treatise on White Magic*. 6th ed. New York, NY: Lucis; 1963:565.

53. Joy WB. *Joy's Way: A Map for the Transformational Journey: An Introduction to the Potentials for Healing with Body Energies*. New York, NY: Jeremy P. Tarcher; 1979:8.

54. De Purucker G. *Studies in Occult Philosophy*. Pasadena, CA: Theosophical University Press; 1945:590.

55. Grof S, Grof C, eds. *Spiritual Emergency*. Los Angeles, CA: Jeremy P. Tarcher, 1989.

56. Bragdon E. *The Call of Spiritual Emergency: From Personal Crisis to Personal Transformation*. San Francisco, CA: Harper & Row; 1990:5.

57. Grof and Grof, *Spiritual Emergency*, pp. 2-26.

58. Oberst MT Editorial: our naked emperor. *Res Nurs Health*. 1995;18:1-2.

59. Blecher MB. Gold in Goldenseal. *Hosp Health Networks*. October 1997;71:50-52.

60. Rifaat H. *Integrating Alternative Medicine and Managed Care* (audiotape #320-S3B). National Managed Health Care Conference; 1997.

61. O'Mathúna DP. Postmodern impact: health care. In: McCallum D, ed. *The Death of Truth: What's Wrong with Multiculturalism, The Rejection of*

Reason, and the New Postmodern Diversity. Minneapolis, MN: Bethany House; 1996:58-84.

62. Rosa LA. Therapeutic Touch: skeptics in hand to hand combat over the latest New Age health fad. *Skeptic.* Fall 1994; 3:40-49.

63. Daniels GJ, McCabe P. Nursing diagnosis and natural therapies: a symbiotic relationship. *J Holistic Nurs.* June 1994; 12:184-192.

64. McCabe P. Natural therapies in Australia: a nurse-naturopath's view. *Nurs Pract Forum.* June 1994;5:116.

65. Carpenito, *Nursing Diagnosis,* p. 356.

66. Ibid.

67. Gross, P.R., and N. Levitt. *Higher Superstition: The Academic Left and Its Quarrels with Science.* Baltimore, MD: Johns Hopkins University Press; 1994.

68. O'Mathúna, D.P. Pharmaceutical companies and nurses: prescriptive authority and postmodern advocacy. In: Peppin JF, Mitchell CB, eds. *Pharmaceutical Industry Interactions with Health Care Professionals: A Reader.* Galen Press. In press.

69. Calvert, R. Dolores Krieger, Ph.D. and her Therapeutic Touch. *Massage.* January/February 1994;47:56-60.

70. Farrar, J., and S. Farrar. *A Witches Bible Compleat: Volume 2: The Rituals.* New York, NY: Magickal Childe; 1981.

71. Buckland, R. *Buckland's Complete Book of Witchcraft.* St. Paul, MN: Llewellyn Publications; 1987.

72. EEOC. *Notice.* 1988. N-915.022.

73. Brierton, T.D. Employers'New Age training programs fail to alter the consciousness of the EEOC. *Labor Law J.* July 1992;419-420.

CONTRIBUTORS

James E. Alcock, Ph.D., is professor of psychology at Glendon College, York University.

Paul Bernhardt is a Ph.D. candidate in the Department of Psychology at the University of Utah. He is also a member of the Rocky Mountain Skeptics.

Berry L. Beyerstein, Ph.D., is Associate Professor in the Brain Behavior Laboratory, Department of Psychology, Simon Fraser University, Burnaby, British Columbia, Canada.

Susan Downie was a senior honors student in 1998 in psychology at Simon Fraser University.

William Evans, Ph.D., is Associate Professor in the Department of Communication at Georgia State University. He is a member of the Georgia Skeptics and the Georgia Council Against Health Fraud, Inc.

Saul Green, Ph.D., Professor Emeritus of Biochemistry at Memorial-Sloan-Kettering Cancer Institute, is now president of Zol Consultants, Inc., in New York.

Ray Hyman is Professor Emeritus of Psychology at the University of Oregon and a founder of the Committee for the Scientific Investigation of Claims of the Paranormal. He currently serves on its executive council.

Rosemary Jacobs is a writer living in Vermont.

Paul Kurtz, Professor Emeritus, State University of New York at Buffalo, is publisher of the *Scientific Review of Alternative Medicine.*

Rebecca Long, a nuclear engineer, is President of the Georgia Skeptics and the Georgia Council Against Health Fraud, Inc.

Steven Novella, M.D., is Assistant Professor of Neurology at Yale University School of Medicine.

Dónal P. O'Mathúna, Ph.D., is Professor of Bioethics and Chemistry at Mount Carmel College of Nursing in Columbus, Ohio. He is a Fellow of the Center for Bioethics and Human Dignity in Chicago, and is also on the Board of Governors of the Ohio Council Against Health Fraud.

Arnold S. Relman is the former editor-in-chief of the *New England Journal of Medicine* and professor emeritus of medicine and social medicine at Harvard Medical School.

Lawrence J. Schneiderman, M.D., is Professor of Family and Preventive Medicine and a medical ethicist at the University of California.